"With so much misunderstanding and disagreement on diets and weight loss, David Medansky offers an achievable, realistic, and simple approach for healthy and permanent weight loss that anyone can do."

– Jack Canfield, *New York Times* best-selling coauthor of *Chicken Soup for the Soul®*

Break the Chains of Dieting

9 Fundamental Must Have Principles for Healthy Weight Loss

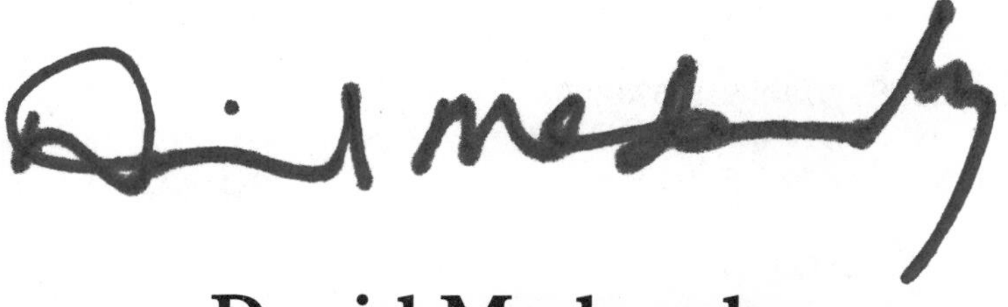

David Medansky

Foreword by Dr. David Friedman, N.D., D.C.
Best-selling, Award-winning author of Food Sanity

Break the Chains of Dieting - 9 Fundamental Must Have Principles for Healthy Weight Loss

Paperback ISBN: 979-8-9850578-0-5
Hardcover ISBN: 979-8-9850578-1-2
eBook ISBN: 979-8-9850578-2-9

Library of Congress Control Number: 2021918337

Front and Back Cover Design: David Medansky assisted by Andrew Hall, President at ThinkandGrowWise.com
Cover Image: Adobe Stock Images by daniilantiq2010
Copyediting: Penny Hill
Proofreading: Patrick Hodges
Interior design: Amit Dey
Published by Spotlight Publishing – https://Spotlightpublishing.pro

Contact:
www.breakthedietchains.com

DISCLAIMER

Before you implement any weight-reduction program, or use any dietary, exercise, or health advice or suggestions from this book, please consult with a medical practitioner or qualified health professional.

All information provided in this book is intended for educational purposes only. Any health or dietary advice is *not* intended as a medical diagnosis or treatment. Statements contained in this book have not been evaluated by the Food and Drug Administration.

The author, publisher, and any other person involved in producing this book disclaim all liability and loss in conjunction with the content provided herein, as well as any and all liability for any products or services mentioned or recommended in this book. The information contained herein is subject to personal research and has been recorded as accurately as possible at the time of publication. Due to possible changes and availability of information provided to the public, you should not take any of the content as a source of reference without further research. The publisher and author are not responsible for any adverse effects or consequences resulting from the use of the suggestions, preparations, or procedures discussed in this book.

If you think you're suffering from any medical condition, then you should seek immediate medical attention.

Results may vary. Causes for being overweight or obese vary from person to person. No individual results should be deemed as typical.

The information contained in this book is based upon the research and personal experience of the author. It is not intended as a substitute for consulting with your physician or other healthcare provider. Any attempt to diagnose and treat an illness should be done under the direction of a healthcare professional.

Break the Chains of Dieting

9 Fundamental Must Have
Principles for Healthy Weight Loss

David Medansky

Foreword by Dr. David Friedman, N.D., D.C.
Best-selling, Award-winning author of Food Sanity

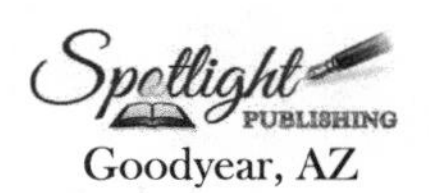

Goodyear, AZ

This book is being given to

Because I care about you and your health,

From:

"When You Eat for Your Health,
Your Weight Loss Journey Will Take Care of Itself."

– David Medansky,
The Overweight Person's Best Friend

THE STARFISH STORY

Adapted from the original by Loren Eisley

An old man was walking on the beach early one morning after a storm. In the distance, he could see someone moving like a dancer. As he came closer, he saw it was a young lady and she was not dancing. Rather, she was picking up starfish and gently throwing them into the ocean.

"Young lady, why are you throwing starfish into the ocean?"

"The surf is up, and the tide is going out. If I don't throw them back in to the water, they will die."

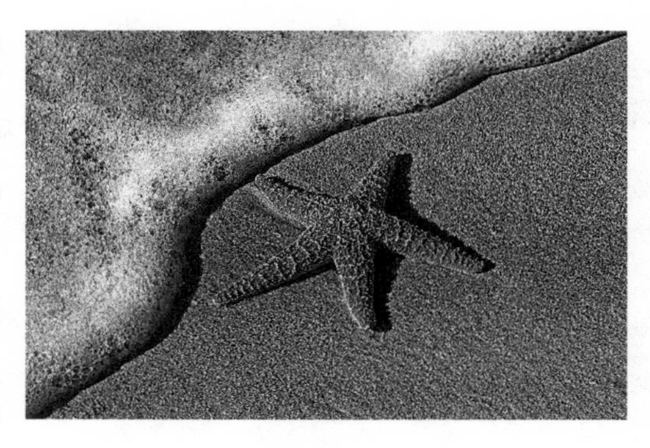

"Young lady, don't you realize there are miles and miles of beach and thousands of starfish? You cannot possibly make a difference!"

After listening politely, the girl paused and then bent down. She picked up another starfish and threw it back into the surf. Smiling, she looked at the old man and said, "I made a difference for that one."

Often, I thought I was too insignificant or too unimportant to make a difference. This story reminded me nothing could be further from the truth.

Today, more than 150 million American adults are overweight. Loosely translated, that is more than 72 percent of the U.S. adult population. What this means for you is if you are at a social gathering with 10 friends, seven of you are overweight, of which 4 are clinically obese. And it is getting worse. Just look around. So, I encourage you to take the time to do something that will make a difference to someone else's life such as sharing the information in this book or giving them a copy. It just might make a difference to your life and theirs.

WHAT OTHERS ARE SAYING

"David… because I found the cover so compelling, I decided to leaf through it, and as I did, I realized it really is a great book… And congratulations for writing such a practical, clearly written, easy to read and compelling book. Well done!"

—Jack Canfield
New York Times best-selling co-author
of *Chicken Soup for the Soul*®

"Have you promised to lose weight before? Did you keep your promise? It's a tough one. Will you keep it this time? We shall see. David Medansky has been where you are, he's been where all of us have been… he lost 50 pounds in four months. So, he can probably assist you with your weight-loss journey… David is a good guy. I know him personally."

—Dean Cain
Superman, *Lois & Clark*

*"**Break the Chains of Dieting** is a book I will recommend to all my past and future nutrition counseling patients. David delivers proven, real-world, every day, common-sense solutions my clients need and seek. Maintaining weight loss is hard for everyone at all phases of life, but David's thought-provoking metaphors, stories, analogies and lessons are spot on to help his readers learn the secrets for healthy and sustainable weight loss."*

—Lisa J. Malone, MS, RDN, CDCES

I love your book. The information is clear, concise, and well packaged. Hopefully, the clarity will cut through the bullshit excuses we all are putting up to avoid addressing the obvious issues.

—Dr. Stephan Neff
Consultant Anesthetist & Director Neff Anesthetic Services Ltd,
Best-selling Author, Speaker and Show host

"If you're ready to take your life and business to better levels and sustain continuous growth and improvement, then you must work with my friend David. Here's the great thing – he focuses on getting you laser focused, cutting you through all of the clutter and inspiring you to produce outcomes!

He's on a mission through his speaking, live events, coaching and online publications to make a HUGE positive difference in the lives of as many people as possible. And he comes from the heart and truly wants to help others. Do yourself a favor and work with David today! You'll be so grateful you did!"

—James Malinchak
Featured on ABCs Hit TV Show, Secret Millionaire,
best-selling author of 20 books,
delivered 3,000+ presentations and 1,000+ consultations

"David Medansky does a masterful job of exposing many of today's diet weight loss myths. If you want to lose weight without going on a diet read ***Break the Chains of Dieting****."*

—Kyle Wilson,
Author of *Success Habits of Super Achievers* and Founder Jim Rohn
International and KyleWilson.com

"Hey David, it's Chris Harrison from The Bachelor," he said in a text message video. *"Your wife reached out to me to let me know that you made some pretty big changes in your life. Actually, you made some small changes that led to a big*

result. So, congratulations – you have lost 50 pounds, a big weight loss, and you've kept it off. She says you made some smart, small decisions that have led to a big change in your persona and your attitude. That is a huge move especially given the times we are in during this pandemic that makes it easy to make some bad choices. So, anybody that is making some positive moves right now, that is a good thing. Congratulations on the book as well. And thanks for being a part of Bachelor Nation.

—Chris Harrison

Host of the ABC reality dating television show,
The Bachelor

I think about David Medansky losing 50 pounds and how it gave him the passion to help other people to lose weight. David helps you overcome the weight-loss challenges you will face by showing you how you can eat within the guidelines of what you are already doing.

—Kevin Harrington

The Original Shark on the hit TV show, Shark Tank, inventor of the infomercial, and responsible for more than $5 billion in sales.

David Medansky's book, **Break the Chains of Dieting** *is insightful with practical, simple solutions for sustainable and healthy weight loss. If you've struggled to lose weight or keep it off, this book is for you. Medansky provides a guide that reminds people what needs to be done to have a healthy lifestyle. He offers suggestions for things you might or might not have known.* **Break the Chains of Dieting** *is a must read for anyone wanting to eat healthier, have more energy, feel better, shed weight, and keep it off, and improve your overall health.*

—Lance Dreher

("Doctor Fitness"), Two-time Mr. Universe, former Mr. America, certified life coach, and National Fitness Hall of Fame Inductee 2019

David Medansky's ***Break the Chains of Dieting*** *provides proven, practical, every day, common-sense solutions interwoven with interesting metaphors, stories, analogies, and lessons for healthy and sustainable weight loss.*

—Forbes Riley
CEO and Creator of SpinGym, National Fitness Hall of Fame Inductee, and TV Health & Fitness Celebrity

When David Medansky asked me to write the foreword to his book If Not Now, When? I was honored and eager to share my message about his work, as he has been a significant part of changing the world's weight mindset in a healthy manner. I think of David as a true innovator and crusader for people's health.

—Lori Shemek Ph.D., CNC
Best-selling author of *Fire-Up Your Fat Burn!* and *How to Fight FATflammation!*

David Medansky exposes many of today's diet and weight loss myths. You'll never look at food the same way after discovering the thought provoking and information depicted in ***Break the Chains of Dieting****. David provides fundamental principles for not only weight loss but maintaining long term success by sharing the secrets of how to master the mind in a world of stress, self-sabotage and worldly distractions.*

—Dr Rachel Smartt ND.
Dr of Naturopathic Medicine, Certified Mind Body Eating Coach, Author, Speaker, Mom of 4, Nutritional Counselor.
SmarttTransformations.com

David is an incredibly thoughtful and caring person. My initial impression from the moment I met him was that he was someone who was genuinely interested in other people and their lives, and he continues to live and breathe that every day. It's something of a rarity these days to find someone who so passionately serves and connects with the people that they're responsible for, but David would definitely be one of those. A nice caveat is that he's also gone through a transformation himself, so he's been through the trenches and has authority on the subject matter at hand.

—Stephen Kung
Business Owner and Associate, World Financial Group (WFG)

David Medansky, *The Overweight Person's Best Friend, is a genuine, caring person who wants to help others succeed along their weight-loss journeys. He has walked the walk, written books, and developed systems to reduce weight and keep it off. He is committed to making people successful because he understands what a drastic danger it is for your health to carry around the extra weight. He's been there. I highly recommend David and his books. He has a great demeanor, is understanding, and keeps you motivated and smiling.*

—Karen Kanefsky
Relationship Marketing Specialist

Last December I turned 63. I felt old, tired, and depressed, and I had been carrying around some extra weight for a few years. I had given up any hope of taking off those extra pounds. I told myself that I was no longer capable of losing that weight, that I was old and that carrying extra weight was all part of being a senior citizen. But David convinced me otherwise. With his help and support I have surpassed my goal of a 30-pound weight loss, and to date I have lost 45 pounds without ever feeling deprived or hungry!!! And I no longer feel like a senior citizen either!! Thanks, David, for helping me feel young again.

—Jan Milliken
Sullivan, Indiana

David knows his stuff. He is very knowledgeable and is very interested in seeing people improve their lives through their health, using science-based evidence and creating better habits. I highly recommend him, and he is always willing to take the time to discuss any challenges or sticking points that I had. He knows his stuff. Thank you, David, for changing my view on life!

—Cory Dunham
CEO of BDB Marketing Design, LLC, Ann Arbor, Michigan

I am fortunate to be David Medansky's friend and client. David's books are remarkably informative. His new book, **Break the Chains of Dieting***, provides easy to follow solutions to lose weight in a healthy way without going on a diet. If you want to feel younger, look younger, improve your overall health, and acquire a new outlook on life, then this book is for you. David Medansky's book teaches you that becoming healthy is simple and something you can do. Be smart and learn the basics of healthy nutritional eating, gratitude, and feeding yourself the fuel your body needs. The information in this book works for me. I am now living a healthier lifestyle and I feel fantastic! My hope for you is you will read this book and share it with others so you too can be on the road to a healthier side of living.*

—David M. Watson
Senior Vice President/General Manager,
Grapes AC Foods - AC Brands

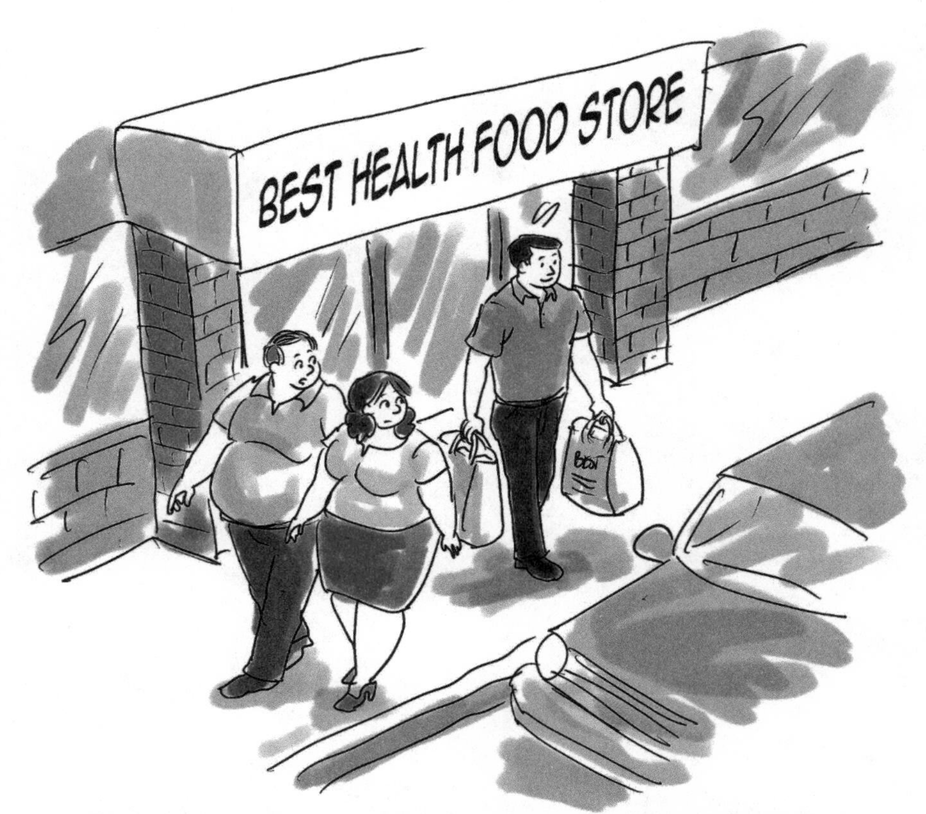

"POOR SCHMUCK, BOUGHT THAT HEALTH FOOD THING HOOK, LINE, AND SINKER."

This book is dedicated to my wife, Debra, who is my angel, and who has had the patience to support me and my endeavors throughout the years. Without her, this book might never have been written.

My mission in writing this book is to help you stop wasting money on FAD (Fat and Desperate) diets that don't work. You can learn how to improve and elevate your own eating routines, behaviors, and habits so you too can lose weight in a healthy and sustainable manner without going on a diet. And, without having to purchase expensive meals, weight-loss supplements, or products, and without needing to count calories, or follow a specific exercise program. My goal is to make an impact by being an example and encourage you and others who want to be healthier.

What is important for you to remember is you can have ***Healthy* Weight Loss Without Dieting.**

The magical ingredients necessary for your successful weight-loss journey are given to you in this book. You just need to follow along. My wish for you is for you to have more vitality, feel better, look better, have more energy, and improve your overall health.

David Medansky

DAILY WEIGHT-LOSS PRAYER

Lord [Universe], thank you for blessing my efforts to lose weight today.

Thank you for helping me to keep the vision of being lighter, healthier, and fitter.

Thank you for watching over me as I seek to monitor all I eat and drink.

Thank you for helping me to enjoy food and to love and care for myself as I lose weight in a healthy and sustainable manner.

Lord [Universe], thank you for giving me energy as I exercise more and become fit.

Thank you for guiding me as I strive to lose weight and blessing my efforts with sustainable weight loss.

Thank you for helping me this day to make healthy choices and give me the strength to fight against destructive cravings that negatively affect my health.

Thank you for helping me to reject any unhealthy behaviors, routines, and habits that give me false comfort.

Thank you for giving me the grace to be strong and encouraging me to keep pushing forward.

Amen.

TABLE OF CONTENTS

FOREWORD

by Dr. David Friedman, N.D., D.C.
Author of the international award-winning number one best-selling book, *Food Sanity,* and host of *To Your Good Health Radio* on Radio MD Podcast

Every day in my clinic, I see patients that are frustrated because they can't lose weight. Many of them blame their family tree and believe they were simply "born to be fat." The truth is that you can't blame your genes on why you can't fit into your jeans. Just look at old photos of your great-grandparents. Only 3% of people living in the early 1900s were considered overweight. Today that number is 70%!

So, if your great grandparents didn't have a weight problem, how can you blame them for yours? The good news is that your biography is not determined by your ancestor's biology.

No matter how many pounds you need to lose, or how much you've neglected yourself, the body has an amazing innate ability for rejuvenation. Every 120 days, new blood cells are formed, which transports oxygen to all of your body parts. The epidermis, or surface layer of the skin, is renewed every twenty days. The cells of your intestines renew every three days. So even if you've consumed daily junk food for twenty years – you get a do-over! It's never too late to make a change and undo the damage that has taken place. Think of your old habits as if they were an image on an Etch a Sketch. Just shake it, and the slate is clean.

But when it comes to achieving permanent weight loss, why is it so difficult? We have access to more gyms, diet books, weight loss programs, health food stores, fat-burning shakes, meal replacements, and supplements than ever in history; yet almost three-quarters of Americans remain overweight or obese. Everyday millions of people go on a keto diet, paleo, Atkins, Whole30, intermittent fasting, or a plant-based diet with the hopes of finally losing those extra pounds. Expensive programs like Jenny Craig, Weight Watchers, and Nutrisystem have never been more popular!

Unfortunately, despite all the time and money being spent on losing weight, the results are usually just temporary. In fact, over 80 percent of dieters regain all the weight they lost or more within a year. Even those that have the guidance of A list professional dieticians and world-renowned personal trainers gain their weight back. This includes contestants of the *"The Biggest Loser"* TV show.

Millions of people watched as they endured an intensive dieting and exercise regimen, which helped them successfully lose between 50-220 pounds. All of this hard work was futile because the majority gained the weight back, and many ended up even heavier. Let's face it, losing weight isn't the difficult part; it's *keeping the weight off!*

David Medansky is not one of these statistics. He was able to lose 50 pounds in four months (25% of his body weight) and *keep it off!* He did not achieve these results by starving himself, or eating things he didn't enjoy, nor did he rely on daily white-knuckle willpower. These are the things that make going on a diet synonymous with suffering. No surprise there, considering the word itself is "die" with a "t."

In *Breaking the Chains of Dieting*, David looks at the bigger picture (pun intended) and shares how it's not necessarily what we eat that's to blame but rather, what's being done to our food supply during the farming, harvesting, manufacturing, and packaging process. These are things that our great grandparents didn't have to worry about.

However, attaining permanent weight loss goes much deeper than focusing just on what you put into your mouth. David's blueprints include proper mindset, stress management, accountability, journaling, and getting deep restorative sleep. I was thrilled to see all these vital pillars for permanent weight loss in *Break the Chains of Dieting*. David didn't just write another "diet book." He has put together a complete success system that will help you finally shed those stubborn, unwanted pounds and become a healthier and better you!

Wherever you are in your journey, if you've found yourself stuck and in need of overcoming stifling weight-loss obstacles, this is the book you've been waiting for.

Dr. David Friedman,
Syndicated TV, and Radio Show Host, International-award winning, #1 best-selling author of *Food Sanity*.

INTRODUCTION

Every human being is the author
of his [or her] own health or disease.

– Swami Sivananda

How successful was the last diet you did? Probably not too good. Let's face it, diets tend to be extreme, temporary, hard to stick with, and potentially dangerous to your health. Have you tried and failed at every diet and weight-loss program, including the big national brands? Conventional diets not only don't work, they also make you miserable, and the word "Diet" has "Die" in it.

It is not your fault you did not lose weight on that diet. The diet is to blame. You did not fail the diet. The diet failed you.

Further, diets are designed to fail. More than 45 million Americans start a diet each year. At any one time, more than 108 million Americans are on a diet. Yet, Americans are getting fatter. The biggest mistake you can make when trying to lose weight: Going on a diet. Some studies show that 95 percent of people fail diets. Dr. Yoni Freedhoff, M.D., however, put it perfectly:

"I don't think 95 percent of people fail diets.
I believe that 95 percent of diets fail people."

Isaiah McCall stated it this way,

> ***"95 percent of people do not fail diets, 95 percent of diets fail people."***

And 95 percent of those who do lose weight on a diet regain it, some even more, within a year. The reason being that the uninformed are being guided by the misinformed. The weight-loss industry is a misinformation machine. Why would I say such a thing? Because Americans spend more than $71 BILLION each year on weight-loss products and services. And still, more than 72 percent of the U.S. population is overweight. Plus, it is getting worse.

Diets are goal oriented. This is one reason why they fail. Because once many people reach their goal, they revert back to their old eating habits. Can you relate to this? Perhaps this is why you keep losing the same 10 pounds over and over again? Saying, "I'm on a diet" carries an inferred message that it is something you will eventually "go off of."

Another reason many popular diets go wrong is because they rely on you to have willpower, self-control, or discipline. For your weight-loss journey to succeed, you must find a way to remove all thinking, all discipline, and all willpower from the equation. If you need to rely on any of that, you are screwed. According to *New York Times* best-selling author Susan Pierce Thompson, PhD, many popular weight-loss programs are fundamentally flawed because they primarily depend on continual willpower and self-control.

The Woman and Missing Keys Story

There is a story about an elderly woman who went for an after-dinner walk. While on her walk she dropped her keys. She kneeled down on the sidewalk under a streetlight and began searching for the missing keys.

Several neighbors and other people passing by offered to help. After five minutes none of them could find the keys. Finally, one passerby asked, "Lady, where exactly did you drop your keys? We've covered every inch around here!"

The woman pointed to an area in the darkness about five feet away.

"Then why in the world are we looking over here?" the passerby asked.

The lady replied, "Because the light is so much better here!"

This story explains why people are overweight and fail to lose weight on diets or keep it off if they do.

Diets are like the streetlight to the woman because like the woman, fat and overweight people are looking for solutions where the light is brightest. People love to believe they can lose weight on the latest trendy diet or magical supplement. I am here to tell you there are no shortcuts to healthy and sustainable weight loss. There is no miraculous fruit, berry, nut, vegetable, or supplement to permanently lose weight. It does not exist. If there was, we'd all be thinner.

There is no lotion to rub on your belly to get rid of fat.

There is no genie in a bottle to grant your wish of being thinner and healthier.

In fact, you should never go on a diet. Instead, change your diet. What this means for you is you must choose to make a conscious decision to improve your eating habits and lifestyle.

Ann Wigmore, a holistic health practitioner and naturopath said, "The food you eat can either be the safest and most powerful form of medicine or the slowest form of poison."

In the movie, *The Equalizer*, Robert McCall (Denzel Washington) tells Teri (Chloe Grace Moretz), when she was wishing to be in a better situation, "Change your world." Now is the time to change your world as it relates to food. What this means for you is that you must change your eating environment: when you eat, where you eat, how you eat, how much you eat, and what you eat. Start now. Because if we put off until tomorrow what we can do today, and tomorrow never comes, that means we will never do what needs to be done. Mark Twain stated it best when he said, "Don't wait. The time will never be just right."

Mark Twain also said, "It ain't what you don't know that gets you into trouble, it's what you know for sure that just ain't so." Be careful of what you think you might know about losing weight because it might not be accurate. Worse, it could be detrimental to your health.

So why is it so difficult for you to lose weight?

Most people fail to lose weight because:

- It is difficult to get started.
- There is no magic formula.
- It is not a quick fix.
- It is challenging to sustain.
- There is no finish line.
- There is no one to hold you accountable.
- Even if you know ***what*** to do you might not know ***how*** to do it.

And, with all the information available about dieting and weight loss, who or what do you believe to act upon?

Time to ACT

Hopefully, by now, you understand that wanting, wishing, hoping, or praying to lose weight is not going to produce results.

Napoleon Hill once asked an audience, "What is the average number of times that a person tries to achieve a new goal before they give up?" After several guesses from the audience, he answered, "Less than one." That is because most people give up before they ever make an attempt. Ask most people "What is your number one priority or commodity?" Most will respond, "My health." Yet, few do anything to maintain or improve their health. The reason being many of you feel you are unable to do so.

Throughout this book you will read stories with lessons about healthy and maintainable weight loss along with solutions. To meet your goals, many of you might need to unlearn what you have learned about dieting, weight loss, and healthy eating. So, from here on out, only positive thoughts. Remember, change is a choice.

So, who the heck is David Medansky and why should you listen to me?

I am not a doctor. Nor am I a mental or health professional. However, I have been where you are. I understand the challenges, frustration, and obstacles you will face along your weight-loss journey to having a healthy weight and lifestyle.

I wasn't always fat. Maybe some of you were like me: we were fit and trim when we were younger. However, as with most people, life gets in the way, whether it be family or work obligations. Maybe you are like me and stopped exercising. Or, like me, you started eating more fast foods and convenience foods. Perhaps, like me, the weight crept up on you.

Like many of you, I struggled with weight issues and dieting. I went on many different diets looking for the perfect one. However, no matter what I did or what diet I attempted, I failed.

If I did lose weight, I was unable to keep it off. Instead of eating one scoop of ice cream, I'd eat an entire pint in one sitting. Or, I'd consume an entire canister of Pringles. If there was a special buy-one-get-one-free sandwich at a fast-food place, I'd eat both sandwiches. I was disgusted with myself. I couldn't believe my pants size ballooned up.

Then something happened to turn my life around. I dubbed it my wake-up call. In July 2016, my doctor told me that based on my lab results and being significantly overweight, I had a 95 percent chance for a heart attack. He gave me two options: 1) lose weight, or 2) find a new doctor because he did not want me to die on his watch. In most things, I am pleased to be in the 95th percentile – however, not if it meant I was likely to die. Suddenly, my being significantly overweight was more than just embarrassing, it was lethal.

With that sword hanging over my head, during the next four months I shed 50 pounds, nearly 25 percent of my total body weight. More importantly, I have kept the weight off. Now I feel great, have more energy, and have improved my overall health. That is what I want for you – for you to have more vitality, more energy, to feel better, look better, and improve your overall health.

Everyone Will Tell You How to Lose Weight

After I released my unwanted and unhealthy weight, I started re-reading the health books I had read in the 1970s. Books such as *Sugar Blues* by William Dufty, books by Paul and Patricia Bragg, Jack LaLanne, Richard Simmons, and others to improve my eating habits and overall health.

Being a former attorney, I am trained to do research – to sift through information and discern between fact, opinion, and fiction. While doing my research for healthy weight loss, I was overwhelmed and inundated with the amount of information available. Thousands and thousands of books have been written about diet, nutrition, fitness, and exercise. Right now, there are more than 50,000 books available on Amazon pertaining to diet, weight loss, health, fitness, and nutrition. At the grocery store checkout, you'll see hundreds and hundreds of magazine articles written about weight loss, many of them touted on the front cover. Thousands of blogs and articles are available when you search Google and YouTube. Numerous weight-loss programs, both national and local, are advertised on TV and radio.

With all the information out there about dieting, who or what do you believe and act on? How do you choose? One expert will tell you one thing, another will say just the opposite. And a third expert will tell you the other two are both wrong.

My goal in writing this book is to help you sort out the myths from the facts and to be your guide along your weight-loss journey. Rick Frishman, best-selling author, publisher, and speaker usually tells his audience at his *Author 101University* workshops, "A book can change a person's life." It is my sincere hope that this book might improve your life.

I realize the information presented here might not be for everyone. However, you may know someone, perhaps a spouse, a friend, a colleague, an uncle, aunt, niece, or nephew who can benefit from the information. If you do, please share this information. It might just save a life.

THE 9 FUNDAMENTAL MUST HAVE PRINCIPLES FOR HEALTHY WEIGHT LOSS

"Simplicity is the ultimate sophistication."

– Leonardo Da Vinci

B**ased on thousands** of hours of research, I have identified nine must have fundamental principles for healthy and sustainable weight loss. They are:

1. Drink an adequate amount (64 ounces or more) of pure water each day.
2. Avoid processed and manufactured foods, also known as edible products.
3. Eat organic, holistic/whole foods, mostly plants.
4. Eat slowly.
5. Eat small portions.
6. Get adequate sleep.
7. Focus on the food you eat by eliminating distractions that can cause "mindless" eating.
8. Give your body 12 to 14 hours each day to digest and process the food you consume.

9. Keep a positive mindset by focusing on the foods you should eat that are healthy rather than the edible products you crave that are known to be unhealthy. What you focus on expands.

If simplicity is the ultimate sophistication, it makes sense to keep your food choices simple. People who live in the world's Blue Zones (areas of greatest longevity) keep their diets simple by having less than 25 ingredients to prepare all of their meals. What this means for you is you need to keep your food choices simple such as avoiding those "edible products" (processed and manufactured foods) and eat more holistic and whole foods.

1

YOU ARE THE PILOT OF YOUR OWN WEIGHT-LOSS JOURNEY

The most difficult thing is the decision to act.
The rest is merely tenacity."

— **Amelia Earhart,**
First female aviator to fly across the Atlantic Ocean, best-selling author of numerous books

To achieve your weight-loss goals, you must do as a pilot of an aircraft does. That is, you must be prepared to make continual course corrections.

An airplane traveling from Los Angeles to New York will end up 150 miles from its intended destination by being pointed merely one degree off course at the beginning of the flight. However, the average plane traveling from LA to New York will be off course more than 90 percent of the time along its journey. Each time the plane drifts slightly off course, its computerized gyroscope corrects it. The gyroscope recalibrates and corrects the flight path to hold the nose of the plane directly toward its destination.

On your weight-loss journey, you will also be off track much of the time. That is because old habits are hard to break, and new habits are difficult to create. What is important to remember is the key to weight-loss success is to keep correcting your eating behaviors to put you back on track. None of us is perfect. We all make mistakes. Those who succeed learn from their mistakes to improve and get back on course. Those who do not succeed in reducing weight and keeping it off fail to keep correcting their eating behaviors.

Vince Lombardi, legendary head coach of the NFL Green Bay Packers, said, "Don't succumb to excuses. Go back to the job of making the corrections and forming the habits that will make your goal possible." What this means for you is forming good habits is necessary to achieving a healthy weight that you can maintain. If you have a setback, correct your mistake, and keep moving forward to improve your eating habits each day. We all justify and have explanations or reasons for not reducing weight or maintaining it. You'll either have excuses or you'll have results. It's your choice.

What is important to remember is that you will never change your weight and improve your health until you change your daily eating habits. The secret of your weight-loss success is found in your daily eating routines.

A routine becomes a behavior. A behavior becomes a habit. And a habit is something you do every day without thinking about it.

Keep this in mind: your weight is based 100 percent on what you eat and drink. Exercise is for fitness and overall health. People always confuse exercising with weight loss. You can shed weight without exercising. However, you can never exercise enough to overcome poor eating habits. Just ask many of the former contestants on "The Biggest Loser" who have regained their weight.

Exercise, however, is important to be fit and for overall health and wellness. Once you shed many of your extra pounds you will most likely want to be more physically active and begin an exercise program. Thomas Edison said, "The doctor of the future will give no medicine but will interest his patients in the care of the human frame, in diet and in the cause and prevention of disease." Edison was wrong. The future is now, yet we consume more processed and manufactured food products that are scientifically engineered so that we never are satisfied. These food products are addicting and deadly.

More than 70 percent of the U.S. adult population is overweight with 41 percent being clinically obese. And it's getting worse. More people are taking medications for preventable diseases and ailments. It's the new normal. I challenge you to be the exception. It's not about my being right or wrong. It's about what you will do. Will you be a part of the new normal or dare to be different?

You Can Lose Weight and Feel Younger Too

Jan M. had just turned 63. She felt old, tired, and depressed, and she had been carrying around some extra weight for a few years. She had given up any hope of taking off those extra pounds. She told herself that she was no longer capable of losing that weight, that she was old and that carrying extra weight was all part of being a senior citizen. However, I convinced her otherwise. With my help and support she surpassed her goal of a 30-pound weight loss and shed 45 pounds without ever feeling deprived or hungry! And she no longer feels like a senior citizen either. Jan is happy feeling young again.

What this means for you is you might need to shift your attitude to get different results.

2

THE PERCEPTION OF BEING OVERWEIGHT HAS SHIFTED

"Twenty years from now you will be more disappointed by the things you didn't do than by the ones you did do."

– Mark Twain

Americans Are Getting Fatter

Recently, a photo of people at the beach in the '70s was posted on Facebook. What was interesting about the photo was that few, if any, of the beachgoers were overweight or fat. The average weight for men between the age of 20 to 74 in 1960 was 166.3 pounds. In 2002 the average weight of a man dramatically increased to 191 pounds. In 2021, the average weight of a man is 197.9 pounds. Meanwhile the average weight of a woman rose from 140.2 pounds in 1960 to 164.3 pounds in 2002 to 168.5 pounds in 2021. Have you noticed a trend?

Socially acceptable body weight is increasing. Why? Because individuals are content with their weight. They are not aware their lifestyles are killing them or that being overweight has severe health-related consequences. And, if they are aware of the negative health consequences from poor eating habits, they don't care. They are less motivated to shed those unhealthy pounds now. An acquaintance of mine asked me how many people would rather die than give up their fast foods and "junk" foods. I told him I did not know. To which he responded, "You should research because you might be surprised." He was right.

What I learned is it is difficult to give up unhealthy habits. It's like a smoker knowing cigarettes can cause lung cancer, yet not wanting to quit smoking. Or, an alcoholic knowing drinking damages the liver, however, not wanting to forego the booze. Let's face it, it's easier to keep eating the same unhealthy fast foods and snacking on junk food than to prepare healthy, nutritious snacks.

Many people also avoid exercising or doing any physical activity. Today, both kids and adults would rather sit and play video games on their phones, tablets, or computers than move around. Virtual reality technology is replacing many sports such as tennis. You can play tennis with a professional without going to the tennis court. Technology has made it such that you can change the channel on your television by a remote so that you do not need to get up. Not to mention that subscription channels play programs without commercials. What this means is that you no longer need to get up from the couch. You can sit for hours without moving. Let's face it, it takes less effort to keep doing the same thing than to make a complete lifestyle change.

Reducing weight is so hard that many people simply don't want to make any effort whatsoever. Good intentions are ineffective and meaningless. However, it is not about the weight so much as it is about your health.

If you want to grasp the concept of what extra weight is doing to your body, try this simple exercise. Carry a one-gallon jug of water in each hand for as long as you can. A one-gallon jug of water weighs approximately 8.36 pounds. In other words, you're lugging around almost 17 pounds of extra weight. After you put the jugs of water down, notice how much lighter you feel. Imagine how much better you'd feel if you lost 20 pounds.

You need to stay conscious of your own weight and the consequences of excess weight because, as I noted above, self-perceptions are changing because it is so common to be overweight or obese. So many people are overweight that we lose perspective. You see so many other people heavier than you that you think you're fine because you're thinner. You're wrong. You're both overweight.

That's a consequence of America's obesity epidemic: the perception of what is normal has shifted. Josh Steimle in his article, *Why Americans are Fat, and the Simple Yet Difficult Solution*, wrote, "...although I didn't think I was *that* fat, because I could see a lot of people around me who were a lot fatter. A LOT fatter. But I was fat enough to feel terrible about myself all the time." Can you relate to Josh?

That reminds me of a story. Some friends were having dinner with us one evening. John mentioned he was going to attend his 50-year class reunion. He and his kids had just finished browsing through his high school yearbook when one of the kids said, "Hey, Dad, can we see that again?"

"Sure. Why?" John replied.

His son opened the yearbook and flipped through it. As the pages cascaded, his son pointed out an interesting observation. "Dad, did you notice that all your high school classmates were thin? There aren't any fat kids."

"No, not really."

Lyle chimed in, "Now that I think about it, there weren't any overweight kids in my high school either."

Afterwards, I went back home to look through my high school yearbook. Wow, what a revelation. There were only a handful of heavy-set kids, none whom I would consider overweight.

Yet, today, many children in grades K through 12 are overweight; some are obese. Think about how that affects self-perception. Sometimes it takes someone to point out the obvious.

Can you relate to this story?

Unfortunately, overweight or obese adults incorrectly believe that their bodyweight is just fine. It's a vicious cycle. As more individuals become obese, more of them are fine with being overweight, they see others with larger bodies, and they become less motivated to shed the extra pounds. Being overweight is the new normal.

In this politically correct society, many people believe you shouldn't do or say anything to make overweight people feel uncomfortable. Even physicians walk a fine line. They don't want patients to have unhealthy bodies but haven't figured out how to make them understand they need to get rid of weight without offending or appearing insensitive.

Today's doctors don't want to intervene. The amount of effort required to understand the patient's needs for weight reduction is more than many doctors are willing to put forth. Instead, they're content to write you prescriptions for medication and manage symptoms rather than address your underlying issues. It is much easier and more profitable for them to prescribe medication than take the time to help a person change their lifestyle.

Some of these same physicians are overweight themselves and don't see a need to help their patients.

While vacationing with my wife in Costa Rica, I met an overweight doctor we'll call Randy. He boasted that most of his patients weighed 300 to 400 pounds.

He had to shed 80 pounds before his orthopedic surgeon would do his hip replacement because he had too much fat. He was still 100 pounds overweight. In other words, Randy weighed 180 pounds more than what is considered healthy.

Randy told tell me that when you get to be his age, money isn't as important as lifestyle. I looked at Randy and said, "I understand."

To which Randy replied, "How could you? You're nowhere near my age."

"Yes, I am," I retorted.

Randy said, "I'm 58. How old are you?"

I replied, "63."

Randy shook his head and walked away. That was the last time I saw him.

Approximately 61 percent of nurses in the U.S. are overweight or clinically obese. And we wonder why there's an epidemic of people being overweight? Perhaps we should listen to Robert Kiyosaki who said, "Stop taking advice from people more messed up than you."

3

NO ONE IS BORN OVERWEIGHT OR FAT

"If you don't like the road you're walking, start paving another one."

– Dolly Parton,
Iconic singer, songwriter, author, actress,
businesswoman, and humanitarian.

No one is born overweight. Being overweight is a learned response. You learned your eating habits by modeling or mimicking your parents, grandparents, friends, co-workers, relatives, and others.

The Pot Roast Story

A young woman was hosting a dinner party for her friends. She served a delicious pot roast. One of her friends enjoyed it so much that she asked for the recipe. The young woman wrote it down for her.

Upon reading over the recipe, her friend inquired, "Why do you cut both ends off the roast before it is put in the pan?" The young woman replied, "I don't know. I cut the ends off because I ***learned*** this recipe from my mom and that's how she has always done it."

Her friend's question got the young woman thinking. The next day she called her mom to ask her: "Mom, when you make the pot roast, why do you cut off the ends before you put it in the pan and season it?" Her mom quickly replied, "Because that is how your grandma always did it and I ***learned*** the recipe from her."

The young woman became more curious. So, she called her grandmother and asked her the same question: "Grandma, I sometimes make the pot roast recipe that I ***learned*** from mom which she ***learned*** from you. Why do you cut the ends off the roast before you prepare it?"

The grandmother thought for a while, because it had been a long time since she made the roast herself. After a moment she said, "I cut them off because when I was first married, the pan I had back then was too small. The roast was always bigger than the pan, so I had to cut the ends off to make it fit."

This is a great story since it teaches us that we do so many things without thinking about why we are doing them because that is how we were taught and how we have always done them. We rarely, if ever, question the reason or rationality of what we might eat or why we might prepare our meals a certain way.

This story demonstrates that before change can happen, you need to gain awareness of why you are doing what you are doing. For many of you, some of your eating behaviors were ***learned*** a long time ago because that is how your parents, grandparents, relatives, or friends ate. An acquaintance of mine, John Canida, calls this "Dietary Duplication."

For your poor eating habits to improve and change, you first need to figure out or analyze why you like or dislike certain foods and beverages. If you drink soda or diet soda, ask yourself why. If you order certain toppings on your pizza, ask yourself why. Do you eat while watching TV, while driving, or at your desk while working? If so, who did you learn this behavior from? Maybe you are mimicking a fellow student, roommate, co-worker, or your parents.

Once you understand why you eat a certain way or what you eat, then change can begin.

John Wooden, legendary UCLA basketball coach said, "When you improve a little each day, eventually big things occur. When you improve conditioning a little each day, eventually you have a big improvement in conditioning. Not tomorrow, not the next day, but eventually a big gain is made. Don't look for the big, quick improvement. Seek the small improvement one day at a time. That's the only way it happens - and when it happens, it lasts." What is important to remember is that Jenna Wolfe, journalist, and personal trainer said, "You did not gain all your weight in one day; you won't lose it in one day."

Patterns of action are like habits. They are done automatically – the things we do without thinking. Sometimes we don't realize what we are doing. We all have patterns for how we eat.

Begin to track the food you eat and the beverages you drink. Nothing too detailed, just some notes. After a few days, see if there are any patterns or correlations to ***what*** you eat, ***when*** you eat, ***where*** you eat, ***why*** you eat, and ***how*** you eat. Then you can begin to self-evaluate to determine what you can do to improve your daily eating habits based on the principles you will learn in throughout this book.

Exercising to Lose Weight Is a Myth

Exercise is not the best way to lose weight. Exercise is to get in shape and improve your overall health. Exercising to lose weight is a myth. Here is why. Most people overestimate how many calories they burn during a workout and underestimate how many calories they consume. Plus, most people tend to eat more when they exercise because they are hungrier.

Fat and muscle weigh the same. However, fat takes up more space than muscle. What this means for you is when you burn fat and increase muscle mass, you either won't lose weight or you will gain weight. Would this frustrate you if you put in the hours of exercising thinking you are losing weight only to see the scale read the same or more? For most people it becomes extremely discouraging, and then they quit.

A client of mine, David Watson, experienced this frustration. During one of our coaching and accountability telephone calls, David expressed his disappointment of not losing weight during the first few weeks of the program. He had modified his eating habits and lifestyle. However, the number on the scale remained the same.

In talking with David, he told me he had started walking about five miles each day, was riding his bicycle, and exercising more. I asked him how his clothes were fitting. David replied that his clothes were loose. He also mentioned that other people were noticing that he looked slimmer.

I explained to him that fat takes up more room than muscle and that he should not be frustrated with the scale. That his clothes will tell him everything about being thinner. After a few more weeks, the scale did start to show a lower number.

What is important to remember is that many people, maybe yourself, set expectations about the number on the scale, and when those expectations are not met, they quit – give up. This might explain why people who make New Year's resolutions to exercise and lose weight stop after a few weeks. Many fail to keep up their workouts because they are not seeing immediate results.

According to Darren Hardy, *New York Times* best-selling author of *The Compound Effect* and world-renowned success mentor, 100 percent of your weight issues is determined by what you put into your mouth. According to Darren Hardy, you don't need to follow a specific exercise program to lose weight.

The Scale Is a Poor Indicator of Your Health

One of the most asked questions is, "How much should I weigh?" or "What is my ideal weight?"

The simple answer is there is no ideal weight. However, according to Dr. Mehmet Oz, as a general rule, your waist size should be one-half of your height. In other words, if you are 5'8" (68 inches), your waist size should be 34 inches or less. If you are 6'0" (72 inches) your waist size should be 36. What is important to remember is a number on the scale does not indicate your "health." Just because a person is thin does not equate to them being healthy.

Scales were available to many doctors and hospitals in the 1870s. However, a patient's weight was not included as part of evaluations. In the early 1900s, mechanical penny scales were mostly for amusement. Put in a penny, find out your weight. They were available in many public places such as drug stores, train stations, grocery stores, just about anywhere you would find a vending machine because they were so profitable.

The home bathroom scale became available to purchase in 1913. The cost was about $10. With the advent of an affordable home scale, weighing yourself went from public to private.

So, how did the number on the scale become so prevalent? Blame the life insurance companies. According to sociologist Amanda Czerniawski, PhD, "Life insurance companies gave Americans the tools to figure out, okay, you're measuring yourself with these scales – now what does that mean?" The life insurance companies used internal height and weight tables to assess the mortality risk of potential insured clients. It is important to understand that it was George R. Shepherd, the medical director of the Connecticut Mutual Life Insurance Company, who first standardized the height and weight actuarial tables, not the medical profession. Prior to Shepherd's standardization, insurance companies used their own version of "average" to determine risk.

Shortly after World War I, life insurance actuaries began lowering the weights printed on the tables from "average" to those they determined were more desirable.

It was during World War II that Metropolitan Life Insurance Company published one of their weight tables. Specifically, it was a table of "ideal weights" for women. The release of this information was so well received by the public, the next year, Metropolitan Life published their "ideal weights" for men. Metropolitan Life ultimately changed "ideal weights" to "desirable weights." The Metropolitan Life Insurance Company remained the prominent authority on American weight until the Body Mass Index (BMI) became the preferred standard around 1985.

Unfortunately, too many people rely on a BMI as a method to determine a perfect weight. Body mass index measures a person's height in relation to their weight. It is not, however, a perfect measurement.

Research has demonstrated errors occur attempting to identify a normal weight range.

Your ideal weight depends on several factors such as your body composition, height, age, genetics, weight, frame size, gender, bone density, body fat distribution, and muscle-to-fat ratio.

Further, BMI fails to indicate a person's healthiness and overall well-being. As an example, just because a person is thin does not mean they are healthy. A thin person might appear fit, yet they might be ill and suffering from poor eating habits, a drug issue, or a fad diet lacking in proper nutrition. Nor is it a good indicator for cardiovascular disease.

In February of 2017, Bob Harper, the fitness idol from *The Biggest Loser*, suffered a near fatal heart attack while working out at the gym. It seems unfathomable that Harper would be susceptible to a heart attack. However, as Harper learned, being healthy is more than being fit and trim. It's about balance and providing your body with proper nutrition.

The BMI doesn't distinguish between a couch potato and a body builder. While BMI is good to study population obesity statistics, it should never be used for determining an individual's overall fitness.

Even the mathematician Adolphe Quetelet, who created the mathematical formula used for the BMI, warned against using it as an indicator for an individual's health. More than 50 million Americans have been inaccurately labeled as obese or overweight based on BMI.

The bottom line is each person's ideal weight will be different because there are too many variables to factor in when calculating an ideal weight. It doesn't exist.

4

WHICH WOLF WILL WIN?

"Weight loss doesn't begin in the gym with a dumbbell; it starts in your head with a decision."

– Toni Sorenson,
Best-selling author

A Cherokee elder was teaching his young grandson about life. "A fight is going on inside of me," he said to the boy. "It is a terrible fight, and it is between two wolves. One is evil. He is anger, envy, sorrow, regret, greed, arrogance. He is self-pity, guilt, resentment, inferiority, lies, false-pride, superiority, self-doubt, and ego.

"The other is good. He is joy, peace, love, hope, serenity, humility, kindness, benevolence, empathy, generosity, truth, compassion, and faith.

"This same fight is going on inside of you and inside every other person, too."

The boy thought about it for a moment and then asked his grandfather, "Which wolf will win?"

The elder simply replied, "The one you feed."

When it comes to your health, eating habits, lifestyle, and food choices, which wolf is winning? Let's begin with the fundamental principles for healthy and sustainable weight loss so you can start to improve your eating and drinking habits to feed the "good" wolf.

THE FIRST PRINCIPLE FOR HEALTHY WEIGHT LOSS

The first principle for healthy weight loss is to drink an adequate amount (a minimum of 64 ounces or more) of pure water each day. However, depending on your body weight, it is recommended you drink one-half of your weight in ounces of water. For example, if you weigh 200 pounds, drink 100 ounces of pure water, which is approximately twelve 8-ounce glasses.

Our bodies are made up of 60 to 70 percent water. Not soda, diet soda, fruit juice, or fruit flavored beverages; pure water. You wouldn't give your dog, cat, or other pets soda or diet soda to drink. Of course not.

Do you drink a minimum of 64 ounces of pure water each day? Probably not. How do I know this?

Because researchers found that more than 70 percent of the U.S. population suffers from chronic dehydration. What this means for you is that seven out of ten people do not drink enough water. If you do nothing else, at least drink more *pure* water.

Americans are addicted to soda and diet soda. The average American drinks about 45 gallons of soda each year. What this means is the average American will have about 375 pounds of soda pass through their bodies each year. Americans spend more money on soft drinks than any other beverage.

Did you know that much of the time when you think you're hungry, you're thirsty?

This could be one reason most of us eat too much. We should be drinking more *pure* water.

What do I mean by pure water?

Pure water, in my opinion, is distilled water, water processed by reverse osmosis, or spring water. It is not the processed flavored waters. There is debate and dispute as to which is better between distilled water, reverse osmosis water, and spring water. I'll leave it up to your preference.

You should drink water at room temperature because it is helpful in soothing and activating your digestive tract, improves circulation, aids in the digestive process, helps relieve constipation, flushes out toxins from your body, and much more. Also, drinking warm water first thing in the morning might help you to lose weight because it could jump-start your metabolism.

Cold water, on the other hand, can be detrimental because it can prevent your body from absorbing vitamins, minerals, and other nutrients. Your body's natural temperature is between 98.6- and 100.8-degrees Fahrenheit. When you drink a cold beverage, your body needs to exert a lot of energy to regulate your core temperature. This diverts energy away from the energy needed to digest your food and absorb nutrients. However, some experts believe you should drink cold water after exercising or other strenuous physical activity because it helps lower your body's core temperature quicker.

Cold water has been shown to increase your risk for headaches. According to a 2001 research study, drinking cold water was twice as likely to induce a headache in women who experienced migraines. Have you ever had "brain freeze" when you ate or drank something cold too quickly? Ouch!

Cold water (or any other cold beverage) may contain ice made from contaminated water. Recent studies found that the ice made in your freezer, store bought, or in beverages from restaurants, is full of bacteria, some of which is unhealthy.

Speaking of contaminated water… Is the water you're drinking safe?

Are you sure?

Because there could be contaminants in your drinking water that have been connected to gut issues, weight gain, food intolerance, autoimmune disease, and cancer.

Academy award winning actress Julia Roberts portrayed Erin Brockovich in the critically acclaimed film, "Erin Brockovich." In the movie, Pacific Gas and Electric Company (PG&E) was exposed for contaminating the water supply in Hinckley, California with chromium

6 and other toxic chemicals. Despite the negative publicity and a $333 million class action settlement in 1996, the problem still exists in 2021. And it's gotten worse.

Many Americans who drink tap water are unknowingly getting a dose of industrial or agricultural waste products connected to cancer, brain and nervous system damage, fertility problems, hormonal disruption, and child-development deficiencies. As of January 6, 2021, chromium 6 and other toxic chemicals were found in more than 200 million homes in all 50 states. This is the disturbing truth documented by Environmental Working Group's (EWG) Tap Water Database. EWG's water database is the most comprehensive and complete source available on the quality of the U.S. drinking water. EWG collects and analyzes data from approximately 50,000 public water utilities.

The bulk of the U.S. drinking water supply get a passing grade from federal and state regulatory agencies. The Environmental Protection Agency (EPA) labels many of the contaminants in our water "within safe limits." Here's the fallacy.

The average person drinks one to two glasses of water each day. More than 70 percent of the U.S. population suffers from dehydration. However, others, like me, drink eight to ten glasses of water each day.

What this means for you is if your neighbor next door drinks one to two glasses of water per day and you're drinking ten glasses, you're drinking five times as much water as your neighbor. Do you really feel it's fair for the EPA to say that toxic chemicals in your water are "within safe limits?"

What is important to remember is that many of these toxic chemicals, such as perfluorooctanoic acid (PFOA) and perfluorooctanoic sulfonate (PFOS), accumulate in the body every time you consume them. Perfluoroalkyl substances are *not* naturally found in the environment. In other words, these are man-made contaminants. They are used for making such things as waterproof materials, paper packaging, fabrics, grease and stain resistant products, and firefighting foam.

What happens after consuming these "within safe limits" chemicals after two years? After five years? Or, after ten years?

In this situation, drinking water that contains chemicals within seemingly inconsequential "safe limits" consistently over a long period of time can result in you contracting chronic diseases and illnesses. You just won't know about these dangerous and harmful chemicals building up in your body until it's too late. Research suggests that continued exposure to low levels of PFOA in drinking water may result in harmful and potentially dangerous health effects.

Still not convinced your water might not be contaminated? Water Quality Association Deputy Executive Director Pauli Undesser said, "It is important for consumers to know that public water systems are *not* required to test and monitor for PFOA and PFOS." The EPA has ***not*** added a new contaminant to the list of regulated drinking water pollutants in more than 20 years. What this means for you is that there are no legal limits for more than 160 unregulated pollutants the tests detect in the nation's tap water.

There is a scene at the end of the movie *Sahara* where a U.S. undercover agent pretending to be a waiter pours a glass of water for the snotty English businessman Yves Massard (Lambert Wilson) from what appears to be a harmless bottle of water. The water, however, is the same contaminated water Yves Massard created with his illegal dumping of industrial toxic waste. Why is this scene in the *Sahara* movie so important? Because in the summer of 2015, high levels of lead were found in the drinking water of Flint, Michigan. The water was deemed safe to drink by federal and state regulators. The contaminated water was discovered only because a worried mother contacted the Environmental Protection Agency (EPA) after her child got sick. Just because you are unable to see contaminants does not mean they aren't present.

More than 250-plus contaminants were detected in water samples that are considered perfectly legal under the Safe Drinking Water Act or state regulations. *However, the level of these 250-plus contaminants are above levels scientific studies have found to cause health risks*. So, let me be clear about this. The government tells you water that contains more than 250 toxic chemicals is safe to drink, yet there is scientific evidence that the same water causes health risks. This is one reason chronic diseases and illnesses in the United States are on the rise.

If you think buying bottled water is safe, think again. Americans spend almost $17 billion each year on bottled water believing it's safe. However, the federal government does more testing and quality control on tap water than on bottled water.

Many brands of bottled water will mislead you and fool you into thinking their water is from underground springs or glaciers. It's B.S.! They are from municipal tap water. This includes two of the most popular brands, Aquafina, manufactured by PepsiCo, and Dasani, produced by Coca-Cola.

Who would have imagined that plain (not to be confused with pure) water with zero calories, zero carbs, zero fat, and zero sugar could be causing you to gain weight? Unfortunately, it is true.

Research shows 80 percent of all diseases are related to our dietary behaviors and habits. This does not include the chronic illnesses correlated to our water intake, or lack thereof. Industrial chemicals are dangerous. They don't belong in our water.

For men, the water you're drinking might be the cause for low testosterone, low sperm count, or man boobs. The endocrine (hormone) damaging chemicals found in drinking water could be the culprit.

Are you among the 30 million Americans suffering from a thyroid issue? Is your doctor telling you this is the reason for your weight gain or inability to lose weight? It might be your water causing your weight issues.

According to the *Journal of Endocrinology*, "A very low dose of endocrine disrupting chemical exposure can have potent and irreversible effects. Research shows that the hormonal system is easily disrupted by a very minimal amount of these chemicals. They can have a negative effect on humans at very low dosages of parts per billion." (*Endocrine-Disrupting Chemicals and Public Health Protection: A Statement of Principles from The Endocrine Society*, published online June 25, 2012.) That means that the government agencies' statement that the amount of these endocrine-disrupting chemicals found in our drinking water is so low that they're

OK to consume, they are wrong. And for some of you it means they're "dead" wrong.

So, what can you do to protect yourself from drinking contaminated water? One suggestion is to invest in a water filtering system (not to be confused with a water filter) that removes these chemicals and heavy metals. However, it should not be just any water filtering system. It needs to be a six-phase reverse osmosis system with re-mineralization.

There are several reverse osmosis systems with seven phases and ultraviolet (UV) light bulbs on the market. These are not recommended because the UV light can heat the water to extremely hot temperatures. The high temperatures can weaken or loosen the fittings. Also, make certain the system has an NSF certification for removal of substance on the label.

Once you have your reverse osmosis system operating, you can use a stainless-steel bottle, a durable BPA-free bottle, or a glass bottle to bring your water with you when you're not at home.

5

SUCCESSFUL AND MAINTAINABLE WEIGHT LOSS REQUIRES A SYSTEM, NOT JUST A GOAL

"A weight-loss goal without a proven process or system is just wishful thinking."

– David Medansky,
The Overweight Person's Best Friend

A goal is an explicit idea of what you want the end result to be. It does not provide you with a plan of action to get there. W. Edward Deming said, "A goal without a method is nonsense." Make certain you have a method to achieve your weight-reduction goal. A motivational meme said, "A goal without a plan is just a wish." Individuals who have successful weight-reduction regimens take the time to create a clear plan. Attempting to reduce weight without a plan is like going from A to Z without stopping in between.

Have you set a weight-loss goal without having a proven, reliable plan or system to accomplish it?

A system creates new eating routines which then become new behaviors and eventually new habits. And your new habits become a lifestyle. You can never own your weight-loss success. You can only rent it. And the rent is due every day in the form of the food and beverage choices you choose to eat and drink.

A life coach or personal trainer knows the importance of goals. They give something to aim for, to achieve, and a way to measure it. For weight-reduction there are two ways to measure your success: 1) the dreaded scale or 2) your clothes to tell you how you're doing.

The simple process to reduce weight is 1) decide to commit to reducing weight, 2) plan how you're going to achieve it, i.e., have a system, and 3) measure your results along the way. Because what doesn't get measured doesn't get done.

Decide your total desired weight-reduction goal and work toward achieving it in increments. People who are successful at reducing weight are very clear about their intentions. Those who fail are generally vague or uncertain. For example, if you decide to reduce your overall weight by 35 pounds, set a target to lose, on average, three pounds each month for 12 consecutive months. Achieving the smaller objectives does three things:

1. Provides a systematic process
2. Creates a sense of accomplishment
3. Gives you small victories to celebrate

Achieving results, no matter how small, helps to keep you on course and encouraged to stay motivated to shed weight.

> How do you eat an elephant? One bite at a time.
>
> How did you gain your weight? One bite at a time.
>
> How will you reduce weight in a healthy and sustainable manner? One pound at a time.

Start small and create a win for yourself. When you do this, you build confidence. With confidence you gain momentum. With momentum, you take more action to move closer to your goal. Nothing sustains motivation more than a sense of accomplishment. Another motivational quote about goals stated, and I'm paraphrasing to remove the vulgar language, "Set goals, stay quiet about them, smash them, clap for yourself, repeat." That's a nice quote; however, it still does not provide a plan to accomplish your goal. Perhaps it should state, *"Set goals, plan how to accomplish them, keep them to yourself, accomplish them, celebrate, and repeat."*

Jim Rohn said, *"Success is not doing a process; it is becoming a process. What you do, what you pursue, will elude you – it can be like chasing butterflies. Success is something you attract by the person you become."* What is important to remember is that a butterfly soars because it trusts the process of change.

THE SECOND PRINCIPLE FOR HEALTHY WEIGHT LOSS

The second principle as it pertains to healthy weight loss is to avoid consuming processed and manufactured foods, also known as edible products. Just as Jacob Marley warns Ebenezer Scrooge in Charles Dickens' *A Christmas Carol*, you are being warned about the dangers of eating manufactured and processed foods as well as other convenience foods. Like Scrooge, you still have time to change.

Ronald Reagan said that the nine words people fear the most are, "I'm from the government and I'm here to help." According to the newly released (2020) U.S. government dietary guidelines, *more than half of U.S. adults have one or more diet-related chronic disease, and emphasize that everyone, regardless of health status, can benefit from changing food and beverage choices to follow healthier diet patterns.* The problem with the new guidelines is that it still allows for 10 percent sugar based on calories. Nutritional values on Nutritional Fact Panels/Labels are based on 2,000 calories per day. However, the average American consumes more than 3,600 calories per day. The food lobby is powerful and influences many of the guidelines, rules, and laws being enacted by Congress. Now you know why people do and should fear government involvement.

Capital One Financial promotes its credit card services by asking, "What's in your wallet?" William Devane in his commercials for Rosland

Capital gold and silver asks, "What's in your safe?" Perhaps the better question to ask yourself is, "What's in your food?"

Do you read the nutritional labels on the cans, packages, or boxes of the food you purchase? If you do, do you understand what you're eating?

Do you read the fine print of those delicious low-calorie recipes in magazines? My guess is that you probably don't because most people won't.

The food industry is, and has been for decades, scientifically engineering the packaged food products you purchase in the grocery store to be addictive. They refer to these enhanced food products as the "Bliss Point."

The "Bliss Point" is a term coined by Howard Moskowitz for how food manufacturers scientifically engineer food to increase the optimization of the food's tastiness and increases your cravings for it. Howard Moskowitz trained in mathematics at Queens College and experimental psychology at Harvard. He was hired by food manufacturers during a 30-year period starting in the 1970s to determine the perfect amount of sweetness, saltiness, texture, and richness for various products. These companies included Campbell Soup Company, General Foods, Kraft, and PepsiCo.

Moskowitz refers to "Bliss Point" as the formulation to create products with the perfect balance of the three main components our bodies crave most – salt, sugar, and fat. It's a complex process pinpointing the exact combination of ingredients that flash our neurological pleasure zones so that we never get the "satisfaction" signal that tells us to stop eating. Like the Rolling Stones, you can't get no satisfaction.

The biggest hits – be they Coca-Cola, Doritos, Oreo cookies, M&M's, Prego spaghetti sauce, Pringles, and others – owe their success to complex formulas that pique the taste buds enough to be alluring yet don't have a distinct, overriding single flavor that tells the brain to stop eating. Simply stated, foods are engineered to be so tasty it's hard to resist them. In other words, they are addicting.

Moskowitz said, "I've optimized soups, I've optimized pizzas, I've optimized salad dressings and pickles. In this field, I'm a game changer."

He had no qualms about his pioneering work on discovering the Bliss Point or any of the other systems that helped food companies create the greatest amount of crave.

So, what does this mean for you?

It means food manufacturers are turning you into food junkies with the junk food they are pushing on you just like a dealer pushes illegal drugs such as meth, opioids, and heroin to junkies. Did you know Oreo cookies are more addictive than cocaine? Imagine that. A cookie is more addictive than an illegal drug.

Moskowitz's formulations for optimization of the amount of salt, sugar, and fat in food products is the Bliss Point for consumer satisfaction. Food manufacturers could care less about the negative health impact it has on your dietary intake so long as they earn a profit.

Bliss Point products were so profitable, food companies looked around grocery shelves to see what other products could be enhanced and expand their product lines. Sugar or other artificial sweeteners were added to foods that didn't use to be sweet. Now, bread has added sugar. Some brands of yogurt can taste as sweet as ice cream. Certain brands of pasta sauce have the equivalent amount of sugar in just a half-a-cup serving as a few Oreo cookies.

Consider this. In 1975 the average supermarket carried about 9,000 food products. In 1995, the average was about 35,000 products. Today, the average grocery store carries more than 50,000 products. Now I don't know about you, but I have not heard of that many new fruits, vegetables, berries, or nuts being discovered during this time period. The reason there are so many more food products is from the rapid increase of processed foods with grains and those being chemically engineered.

What does this mean for you?

Nutritionists say this creates an expectation that everything we eat should taste sweeter (or saltier). This is one explanation why kids rebel against eating fresh produce. To them it tastes bitter or sour.

Unfortunately, because of these Bliss Point food products, the human body has evolved to crave foods that deliver just the right amount of saltiness, richness, and sweetness. That's because your brain responds with a reward in the form of endorphins. It remembers what you did to get that reward, and makes you want to do it again.

This is the reason why you want to keep eating your junk food even though you are full. It's an effect run by dopamine and neurotransmitters. Your mind will never be satisfied. You can never get enough – just like a junkie on heroin. Perhaps that's why it's referred to as junk food. Because it makes you a food junkie.

Food manufacturers use combinations of sugar, fat, and salt synergistically because the combination is even more rewarding than any one alone. Their goal is to create products with two or three of these ingredients (salt, sugar, and fat) to target your Bliss Point and optimize your desire to consume more and more of them.

Artificial Ingredients – Also Known as Fake Fat and Fake Sugar

Processed foods now contain chemicals also referred to as artificial ingredients to enhance their flavor and taste. What are some of these artificial ingredients?

- Olean
- Aspartame
- High-fructose corn syrup

Let's start with Olean

What is Olean? Olean, formerly known as Olestra, started out as a drug, and later was developed by Proctor & Gamble to be a calorie and cholesterol-free fat substitute. The Food and Drug Administration (FDA) approved Olestra as a food additive in 1996, concluding that it "meets the safety standard for food additives, reasonable certainty of no harm." However, as it turned out, it is detrimental to your health. In the late 1990s, Olestra lost its popularity due to negative side effects.

Because Olestra adds no fat, calories, or cholesterol to products, it is used in the preparation of otherwise high-fat foods such as potato chips, pretzels, and cookies to lower or eliminate their fat content. Since Olestra is unhealthy for you, food companies are required to put warning labels on the food products that contain it. The FDA mandated health warning label read, *This Product Contains Olestra. Olestra may cause abdominal cramping and loose stools (and leakage). Olestra inhibits the absorption of some vitamins and nutrients. Vitamins A, D, E, and K have been added.*

Proctor & Gamble argued that the label did not accurately communicate information to consumers because it was unlikely that Olestra would cause serious digestion problems. In 1996, the FDA agreed with Proctor & Gamble and stated that the label could be removed. By then, however, the damage from the negative publicity about Olestra had been done.

Undaunted, Proctor & Gamble renamed and rebranded Olestra as Olean. It's still unhealthy for you, yet it is legal in the United States, and it is found in many "fat free" or "light" products. Olean, however, is banned in Canada, China, and the European Union (EU). You should never eat this ugly fat! *What is important to remember is just because a food product is legal does not necessarily mean it is safe for you to consume.*

Products with Olestra/Olean are by far worse than any other fat, carb, or gluten you can put into your body because this additive prevents your body from absorbing any essential vitamins and minerals. Some of the common side effects include diarrhea, cramps, leaky bowel, and gas.

Some of the brands it is found in include:

- Lays Light Potato Chips
- Pringles
- Ruffles
- Doritos

Do you snack on some of these products? Are you snacking on these products right now as you're reading this book?

When Lay's Potato Chips says, "Bet you can't eat just one," it's not a dare. It's a fact!

The FDA, for whatever reasons, still allows Olestra/Olean to be a legal food additive despite its health implications. Keep in mind that

Olestra started as a drug and then became a food additive – an artificial, scientifically engineered food additive.

Finding the Sweet Spot

Aspartame, also labeled as phenylalanine, is another Bliss Point ingredient used in processed foods. Aspartame is one of the most common artificial sweeteners in use today. It is sold under the brand names NutraSweet, Equal, Spoonful, and Equal-Measure.

Do you use these products?

Do you use Stevia? If so, be careful if you purchase Stevia in packets in grocery stores. Most, if not all of them, are a blend of fructose, sucrose, dextrose, and stevia or a variation thereof. Some packages will state it's a blend. Some are deceptive and won't. Be certain to read the nutrition label. In my opinion, the only place you should trust to purchase pure stevia is at Sprouts, Whole Foods, and other reputable health food stores. The only ingredient in stevia should be stevia and nothing else.

Aspartame is used in many foods and beverages because it is 200 times sweeter than sugar. Food manufacturers can use less of it, thereby lowering calories in their products. Plus, it is much cheaper than sugar. The end result is more profits for these companies, all to the detriment of your health.

Aspartame was inadvertently discovered in 1965 by James Schlatter. Schlatter was a chemist at G.D. Searle Company testing an anti-ulcer drug.

Have you notice the similarities between Olean and aspartame?

Both started out as drugs, and both are artificial. That means it is not produced by nature. One of the elements for eating healthy is to eat holistic or whole foods and avoid processed or manufactured foods.

Aspartame, manufactured by G.D. Searle, was approved for use in carbonated beverages in 1983. Monsanto purchased G.D. Searle in 1985 and spun off the aspartame business as the NutraSweet Company. Think about this: Monsanto also manufactures Roundup, Agent Orange, DDT, PCB, and many other insecticides. Speaking of engineered foods, Monsanto was among the first to conduct field testing of Genetically

Modified Crops. They're better known today as GMOs. GMO Foods will soon be called "Biofortified."

Why was the name changed? Because food manufacturers realized that consumers were becoming wise about the dangers of GMOs. This name change is a deliberate fraud perpetuated on you, the consumer. Food manufacturers did the same thing with Monosodium Glutamic Acid (MSG). MSG is a food additive that's been linked to chronic illnesses such as obesity, liver disease, high cholesterol, metabolic syndrome, neurological, and brain health issues, etc. The food manufacturers changed the name of MSG to "Autolyzed Yeast" so people wouldn't know they were consuming MSG.

When aspartame was implicated in serious health issues, some food manufacturers changed the name to "Amino Sweet." Don't be fooled. If Charles Manson legally changed his name to John Smith, he'd still be just as evil. Read labels. However, aspartame is still called aspartame in plenty of products.

Aspartame is now found in thousands of different food products. It's commonly used as a table-top sweetener as a replacement for sugar. It is added to prepared foods and beverages that do NOT require much heating because heat breaks down aspartame.

The primary reason not to drink diet soda is because it contains aspartame. There are 92 documented negative side effects of aspartame. One of them is that it causes people to gain weight – *not* lose it. Aspartame affects your metabolism, so you cannot burn calories. While a diet soda may contain zero calories, it will prevent you from reducing weight, and cause you to gain weight. It also inhibits or prevents your body from absorbing vitamins, minerals, and other essential nutrients. That's why it's dangerous. You are depleting your body of the proper nutrients and it goes into starvation mode, which causes weight gain. Just because aspartame is legal does not mean it's safe. Other reported side effects include, but are not limited to:

- Cancer
- Seizures

- Headaches
- Depression
- Attention Deficit Hyperactivity Disorder (ADHD)
- Weight Gain
- Birth Defects

There is controversy about this sweet deception. You will find a lot of information on the internet about aspartame. Some of these articles indicate that aspartame is safe for you. They have studies to support their claim that no health problems have been linked to aspartame. There are just as many, if not more, articles about the adverse side effects of aspartame.

This is some of what you'll learn reading up on aspartame. A 25-year study found very moderate consumption of aspartame is linked to a 65 percent higher likelihood of being overweight and a 41 percent increased likelihood of being obese. A new study shows it's toxic to your gut and sparks DNA mutations. Aspartame will ruin your health.

Many people turn to Sweet'n Low, Equal, or Spoonful thinking it will help them consume fewer calories, slim down, and lower their risk of developing Type 2 diabetes. However, researchers are now learning that's not the case. Instead, aspartame accumulates in your blood, meaning your body cannot get rid of or eliminate it. This can cause even more severe damage to your blood vessels.

Yet another study has linked artificial sweeteners to impaired glucose response, suggesting they may play a role in Type 2 diabetes and can increase risk for obesity and other related health problems.

Aspartame accounts for over 75 percent of the adverse reactions to food additives reported to the FDA. Many of these reactions are very serious.

Other chemically engineered artificial sweeteners such as Splendid and saccharine are just as toxic and poisonous. For example, saccharine is made from coal tar. Coal tar is a derivative. It is not a food. It is a chemical. Splendid, which is the brand name for sucralose, is a form of sugar made with chlorine. As you know, chlorine is a cleaner.

Sweet Deception

Let's talk about the worst artificial ingredients added to your food: High-fructose corn syrup (HFCS), otherwise known as glucose-fructose, isoglucose, and glucose-fructose syrup.

Do you know why high-fructose corn syrup has so many different names?

It's because food manufacturers know you, as a consumer, are more aware of how bad it is for you. They are attempting to disguise that their products contain HFCS by calling it something else. It's the same.

What is high-fructose corn syrup? HFCS is a sweetener ***processed*** from corn starch. Starches are made from long chains of linked sugars. Manufacturers break down corn starch into sweet corn syrup made of the sugar glucose. Enzymes are added to make the syrup much sweeter.

Why do manufacturers do this?

Because it's much cheaper and easier than producing sucrose, which is ordinary table sugar. The ratio of fructose to glucose is nearly the same as HFCS to table sugar. Both have 4 calories per gram.

Studies show that animals, such as chickens, that eat a high-fructose corn syrup diet gain more weight than those that don't. How many of you are starting to understand that because many chicken breeders are feeding their birds diets high in HFCS chickens are getting bigger and bigger? A plumper bird returns a higher price. It's all about the profit margins, your health be damned.

HFCS was first marketed in the early 1970s by the Clinton Corn Processing Company of Clinton, Iowa. It is composed of 76 percent carbohydrates and 24 percent water. It contains no fat, no protein, and no essential nutrients. One tablespoon has 53 calories.

HFCS is found in sodas, desserts, some breakfast cereals, and elsewhere. It is linked to obesity, diabetes, and even some forms of cancer.

There is a debate as to whether HFCS is unhealthy for you. You can find studies done to support that it's *not* harmful. The question I'll pose to you is if HFCS is not harmful to your health or doesn't have negative side effects, then why go through the trouble of calling it by different names on the Nutrition Facts label?

Avoid anything ending in "OSE." That includes dextrose, sucrose, glucose, fructose, and isoglucose. You get the idea.

More Fake Foods: Meatless Meat, Chicken-less Chicken, Fishless Fish

According to Dr. David Katz, M.D., who refers to Michael Pollan, a simple solution to reduce weight and improve overall health in a sustainable manner is to...

- Eat holistic food
- Not too much
- Mostly plants
- Avoid processed foods, and
- Drink lots of pure water

Sounds simple, yes?

No. Because if it were that simple, everyone would be eating this way. The problem today is the biggest trend in the food industry has nothing to do with organic beef or free-range chicken. In fact, the juiciest burgers you might eat are made of pea protein and other chemicals.

Popular examples of plant-based meat include the Impossible Burger, the Beyond Burger, and the myriad of options now commonly found in the freezer section of the grocery store. Plant-based burgers are now sold in fast-food places such as McDonald's, Burger King, White Castle, Carl's Jr., and other fast-food places. Even prestigious, posh, upscale restaurants are serving the Impossible Burger with their own creative toppings.

Plant-based alternative meats do not only apply to beef. Chicken and sausages are being manufactured to look and taste as close to meat as you can get without harming a chicken (KFC's vegan fried chicken) or pig. While plant-based meat, chicken, and fish are often heralded for tasting and looking like the real thing, many experts are still unsure if they are healthy.

In the 1970s, Chiffon Margarine began running television ads that featured Hollywood actress Dena Dietrich as Mother Nature. Her character's slogan, "It's not nice to fool Mother Nature," became a pop culture catchphrase. Perhaps today's consumer should heed these words as a warning.

These meat substitutes aren't as good for you as you may think. You have to look at the ingredients and nutrition facts to find out exactly what you're eating. It is important to remember that these are still "highly processed" products.

What makes new-age burgers like the Beyond and the Impossible so unique is that they don't use ingredients such as rice, whole peas, beans, tofu, and seitan (wheat gluten) to mimic meat. Instead, these plant-based meat companies introduced a *new* substance, a molecule called "heme." Heme is the key ingredient that's responsible for making meatless products look and taste so authentic, so much like the real thing.

So, what is heme?

Heme is an essential molecule containing iron that is found in the blood of humans and animals. Heme gives meat that metallic flavor, makes it pink, and makes your blood red, too.

However, according to Impossible Foods, soy leghemoglobin (which stands for legume hemoglobin) and is found in soybeans is a protein that contains heme. This "miracle" ingredient is a genetically modified organism (GMO) that's modified and created in a lab by manipulating the DNA of the soybean and adding yeast. In other words, the heme used in plant-based meat alternatives is a genetically modified organism. Some consumers worry about traces of glyphosate in Impossible Burgers, which is made from those genetically modified soybeans.

If you analyze the labels of the Beyond and Impossible burgers, you will see a long list of ingredients, only a few of which are recognizable as whole foods. That is because the main ingredients, pea protein isolates and soy protein concentrates, are extracts taken out of plants in a lab.

They are not whole foods; they are just *part* of a food. Both burgers include coconut and other oils, and each includes a host of ingredients such as methylcellulose, soy leghemoglobin, zinc gluconate, modified food starch, cultured dextrose, and soy protein isolate. What this means for you is the imitation (fake) meat is *not* a holistic/whole food. It is a scientifically engineered food product. Do not confuse real food with food products. There is a difference.

John Mackey, the CEO of Whole Foods Market – which introduced Beyond Meat's first products in 2013 and carries its full line of burgers and sausages along with many other plant-based "meats," recently told CNBC that he believes these products *are not* a healthy choice. Mackey said, "If you look at the ingredients, they are super, highly processed foods." Mackey added, *"I think people thrive on eating whole foods."*

Studies have shown that switching from a meat-based diet to a plant-based diet can have numerous positive effects on your health. However, if you think simply switching from animal-based meat to an alternative plant-based meat *might* give you improved health, you'd probably be mistaken. The more practical solution is for you to add lots of organic vegetables, fruits, and whole grains to your diet. After all, according to Dr. David L. Katz, M.D., a simple solution to reduce weight and improve your overall health is to drink an adequate amount of pure water, eat mostly plants, not too much, and avoid processed and manufactured foods. Keep in mind that these plant-based "meats" are highly processed and manufactured food products. And alternative meat products are more expensive than regular meat products.

On the other hand, this doesn't mean that regular animal proteins are the healthier option. Here is why. Industrial animal meat is treated with chemicals, and it tends to be contaminated with bacteria. The beef industry is known to overuse antibiotics. The overuse of antibiotics in beef has made millions of people antibiotic resistant. Further, most of the cattle, chicken, and pigs are fed corn and soy, which are GMOs.

Conventional wisdom and common sense dictate that organic vegetables, fruits, legumes, nuts, seed, and berries remain the cheapest and most sustainable healthy food choice options.

What's in Your Sandwich?

How many of you make sandwiches to take to work? A sandwich with a few slices of deli meat is a cheap and quick brown-bag lunch. Unfortunately, sandwiches made with deli meat or processed meats have been linked to increased risk of cancer, diabetes, and heart disease.

How many of you are wondering what deli meats or processed meats actually are?

Ham, bacon, pastrami, salami, and bologna are *processed meats.* So are sausages, hot dogs, bratwursts, and frankfurters.

In 2007, a review of 7,000 studies found convincing evidence that high intakes of processed meat increased the risk of colorectal cancer. It was thought that chronic obstructive pulmonary disease (COPD) was primarily caused by cigarette smoking. COPD was the third most common cause of death worldwide in 2010. However, up to one-third of patients who contracted COPD had never smoked. This suggested that other factors were involved. Until recently, little attention had been paid to these other factors, such as diet.

An article published in the *European Respiratory Journal,* Volume 43, Issue 4 published on March 31, 2014, found that a steady diet of processed meats (bacon, gammon, ham, corned beef, Spam, luncheon meat, sausage, meat pies, etc.) was linked with weak lung function, in both males and females. Further, health professionals determined that cured meat consumption was directly related to newly diagnosed COPD cases. And another study in Spain of patients with COPD showed that everyday consumption of cured deli meats exacerbated COPD and symptoms.

In 2015, the World Health Organization classified processed meats as "carcinogenic to humans" and red meat as "probably carcinogenic."

Red meat is any meat from a mammal (for example beef, veal, pork, goat, lamb, and bison).

Another recent study found that people who ate more than 160 grams of processed meat (equivalent to two large Italian sausages or three slices of deli ham and three small hot dogs) each day – versus less than 20 grams – were 44 percent more likely to die early from cardiovascular disease or cancer.

What makes processed meat so unhealthy? For starters, it's a source of saturated fat, the type that raises blood cholesterol. It's also very high in sodium. Four strips of cooked bacon, for example, packs 800 milligrams, more than half a day's worth. And, it has high amounts of nitrates and nitrites.

Sodium nitrates and sodium nitrites are salt compounds that naturally occur in the soil and are in many fruits and vegetables, such as celery, leafy greens, and cabbage. In fact, most of the nitrates we eat come from vegetables and drinking water. When nitrates contact with saliva in the mouth, they convert to nitrites.

Sodium nitrate is added to cold cuts for preservation and to inhibit bacteria growth. Nitrate is converted to sodium nitrite when it connects with bacteria in the meat. Most manufacturers now directly add nitrite to the meat. Nitrates and nitrites themselves do not cause cancer; however, there is concern that they may produce carcinogenic compounds in the body or during processing or cooking.

Frances Largeman-Roth, R.D.N., a nutrition expert and author of *Eating in Color*, says, "We know that when nitrites combine with the amines in meat, they create nitrosamines, which some studies have found to be carcinogenic."

Because consumers are wary, some manufacturers now cure meats with celery powder since celery is naturally high in nitrate. These meats are labeled "uncured" and "celery powder" is in the ingredients list instead of "sodium nitrite."

Cooking meat at high temperatures forms heterocyclic amines, compounds that have been linked to cancer in animals and colorectal polyps in people.

Am I suggesting for you to eliminate eating processed meats altogether? No, of course not! I'll still enjoy bacon with my eggs on occasion or a hot dog. However, it's not part of my normal eating routine. I enjoy them on few occasions, such as at a baseball game or at a friend's BBQ.

So, what are some healthier alternatives for sandwiches? Healthier sandwiches and wraps include tuna, salmon, hummus and veggies, or fresh, cooked poultry. When you're baking or grilling chicken, cook extra for lunches during the week. Or roast a whole fresh turkey breast on Sunday to slice up for sandwiches and salads during the week.

Google or watch a YouTube video on how to make a Mediterranean wrap. Remember, it's more than just the meat. It's about the bread, cheese, mayo, and other condiments that people, such as yourself, like to add to their sandwiches. When you add up all the sodium, fats, sugars, and nitrates from the ingredients in a sub sandwich, club sandwich, or "specialty" sandwich at your favorite restaurant – yikes.

Let's talk about bread, the foundation of every sandwich. White flour, which is used to make white bread, is the absolute worst, since the bleaching process that it undergoes strips away all the nutrients. Consuming white bread can cause a spike in blood sugar, weight gain, and inflammation.

Whole-grain bread, not to be confused with multi-grain, is a much better choice. It's loaded with fiber, healthy plant-based protein, vitamins, minerals, and a variety of phytochemicals that help to improve digestion, reduce inflammation, and lower cholesterol. Whole-grain bread also contains lactic acid, which promotes the growth of good bacteria in the intestines. Rye bread is another healthy option. Research published in the "Nutritional Journal" shows that rye bread can help decrease hunger for up to eight hours.

If you're serious about shedding your unwanted pounds and getting rid of that extra weight, simply avoid eating a sandwich. In the alternative, use Ezekiel bread. Ezekiel bread is a flourless bread made using a variety of sprouted grains. The sprouted grains increase the nutritional value of the bread. And, unlike other store-bought breads that can last on a shelf for months, Ezekiel bread must be refrigerated or frozen because it will otherwise spoil quickly.

Next time you're at a restaurant, check out the menu to see what they state are the calories for each dish. You might be shocked. And that's just the calories. Most places will not provide you with how much sugar, salt, or fat is in an item being served.

If you look at the packaging of processed foods in the grocery store, it will tell you about the low sodium, low fat, low calories, and so forth. However, what they might not tell you, is the amount of carbohydrates or other information that is unhealthy because it's such a large quantity. For example, the front of some spaghetti boxes might state, "0 cholesterol, 0 sodium, low fat or no fat, 0 sugar." And many of you might be thinking "that sounds good." Yes, it does. What they don't tout or promote is it has 42g of carbohydrates per serving. That's more than a typical ice cream sandwich, Häagen-Dazs, or Dove ice cream bar. Those have between 26g and 34 grams of carbohydrates. If you're reducing weight, you need to consume less than 60 grams of carbs per day. What is important to remember is that there is a huge difference between simple carbohydrates and complex carbohydrates.

Keep in mind, it's more than just calories in and calories out if you're attempting to reduce weight in a healthy manner that's sustainable. Achieving and maintaining a healthy weight is about choices. We all have choices. Why wait until you're in a health crisis if it can be avoided?

The American Heart Association recommends eating no more than 2,300 mg of sodium per day (for some groups even less). Unfortunately, we are consuming much more. Kids in the U.S. eat an average of 3,279 mg of sodium per day. Adults average more than 3,400 mg per day.

With cold cuts, the sodium adds up quickly given that just one ounce of deli turkey can have more than 500 mg of sodium. A slice of cheese has 150 mg. Each slice of bread has 140 mg. One sandwich may be close to 1,000 mg of sodium, not including any extra condiments like mustard or mayo. That's almost half of our daily requirement in one part of a meal. Since the mid-1980s medical research has known that 80 percent of the three leading causes of pre-mature death are, 1) overconsumption of processed food, 2) smoking tobacco, and 3) inactivity. Dr. David L. Katz refers to these as the three "Fs."

- Food – overeating processed foods,
- Fingers – used for smoking,
- Feet – lack of walking, running, or other physical activity.

Bliss Point used to create processed foods has caused many of today's chronic diseases. Chronic diseases take life from years, and years from life. Dr. Katz says, "I'm all about adding life to years and years to life."

What is important to remember is that obesity now causes more deaths than smoking.

And four out of every ten U.S. adults are clinically obese.

What does that mean for you?

It means that you're more likely to die from overeating than from smoking. In society today, it's no longer health care – it's disease care. According to the 2017 Bloomberg Global Health Index, the United States ranks 34th in the world for health. The U.S. ranking of 34 out of 163 countries who met the criteria to be evaluated was negatively impacted because of the prevalence of overweight people.

Imagine making some small adjustments to your daily eating routines that you do consistently over a long period of time to give you noticeable results, such as a smaller waistline, having more energy, being able to spend more time with the kids or grandkids and being physically active with them, improving your overall health, and lowering your risk for expensive medical ailments, even death.

Hydrogenated Oil

Hydrogenated oils are vegetable oils whose chemical structure has been altered to prevent rancidity in foods, which increases shelf life and saves money for food manufacturers. The process of hydrogenation involves the addition of hydrogen atoms to the oil's available double bonds. As the level of hydrogenation increases, the level of saturated fat increases and the level of unsaturated fat decreases.

The hydrogenation process converts what are known as "cis" double bonds to "trans" double bonds. During this manufactured partially hydrogenated processing, a type of fat called trans fat is created. Food manufacturers like hydrogenation because it has the technical advantage of making foods solid or partially solid at room temperature. Food companies prefer using hydrogenated oil because it does extend the shelf life of products and save costs. This comes at a cost… to you. Trans fats raise total blood cholesterol levels and LDL and increase your risk for heart disease. There are two types of trans fats found in food: 1) naturally occurring and 2) artificial, where they add hydrogen to the liquid oil (partially hydrogenated oil). In other words, hydrogenated oil is another processed food used in the preparation of what you're being given to eat.

These partially hydrogenated oils block the production of chemicals that combat inflammation and benefit the hormonal and nervous systems, while at the same time allowing chemicals that increase inflammation. This means that trans fats promote inflammation and negatively impact cholesterol levels.

The Harvard School of Public Health notes that trans fats promote immune system over-activity and inflammation and are linked to heart disease, stroke, and diabetes, among other chronic diseases. One 2006 article published in the *New England Journal of Medicine* noted that at that time the average American consumed nearly 5 grams of trans fat per day – an amount that increases the risk for heart disease by approximately 25 percent.

The artificial trans fats are:

- Easy to use.
- Inexpensive to produce – it's cheap. More profits for the food providers.
- Used to increase stability and extend the shelf life of products.
- Used to enhance the texture of food.
- Used by many restaurants and fast-food outlets to deep fry foods because trans fat can be used many times in a commercial fryer.

On the other hand, *fully* hydrogenated oil contains very little trans fats and doesn't have the same health risks as trans fats. Because partially hydrogenated oil contains trans fats, it's best to avoid any food that contains it. Partially hydrogenated oil is found in:

1. Margarine
2. Microwave popcorn
3. Cakes, pies, and cookies
4. Doughnuts
5. Vegetable shortening
6. Packaged snacks
7. Baked foods, especially premade versions
8. Ready-to-use-dough (Thank you Pillsbury Doughboy)
9. Fried foods (onion rings, French fries, fried zucchini)
10. Coffee creamers, both dairy and non-dairy

Partially hydrogenated oil isn't always easy to spot, but there are ways to spot it and avoid it.

Some food labels claim they have no trans fats, but partially hydrogenated oil may be listed as one of the ingredients. It's important to read both the Nutrition Facts label and the ingredients list.

Food preservation goes hand in hand with packaged foods – longer shelf life. Decrease or eliminate your dependency on packaged foods. For example, cook your own brown rice (avoid white rice) or potatoes from scratch instead of purchasing the boxed versions. Yes, it's quicker and more convenient to prepare the boxed version. But this is where you get to choose what you want to put into your body.

Consider baking or broiling your foods rather than frying them. Use heart-healthy oils such as safflower, olive, or avocado oil.

I'm amazed how many people are concerned about air pollution and water pollution but have no qualms about polluting their own bodies.

Consider preparing your own snacks. Some ideas for healthy, great tasting snacks include:

- Raw unsalted nuts such as walnuts, pecans, and almonds
- Carrot sticks
- Celery
- Apples
- Berries such as blueberries, strawberries, raspberries, and blackberries
- Raw cheese (avoid processed pasteurized cheese if possible)
- Plain Greek yogurt without the added fruit. It's best to add your own berries or fruit

"Fitness is like marriage.
You can't cheat on it and expect it to work."

– Bonnie Pfiester,
Certified Personal Trainer, nutrition coach,
TV host, and fitness personality.

6

LOSE WEIGHT ONE POUND AT A TIME

"The people you surround yourself with influence your behaviors, so, choose friends who have healthy habits."

– Dan Buettner,
Explorer, National Geographic Fellow,
New York Times bestselling author of *The Blue Zones*

In the movie *Rocky Balboa* (2006) Rocky tells his son, "Let me tell you something you already know. The world ain't always sunshine and rainbows. It's a very mean and nasty place. And I don't care how tough you are. It will beat you to your knees and keep you there permanently if you let it. You, me, and nobody is going to hit as hard as life. But it ain't about how hard you hit, it's about how hard you can get hit and keep moving forward. How much you can take and keep moving forward. That's how winning is done...

"You got to be willing to take the hits and not pointing fingers saying you ain't where you want to be because of him or her or anybody. Cowards do that and that ain't you. You're better than that!

"Until you start believing in yourself, you ain't going to have a life."

Paraphrasing Rocky, "Stop pointing fingers saying you are not the weight you want to be because of him, her, or anybody. You choose what you put in your mouth. You decide what you are going to eat, where you're going to eat, when you're going to eat, and how fast you will eat. Until you make a commitment to improve your eating habits, you're never going to shed those excess pounds. You are better than that!"

A Frog Story

Several frogs were hopping through the forest when two of them accidentally hopped into a deep pit. The other frogs stood around the pit, and, seeing how deep it was, they told the two frogs that they couldn't help them. There was no hope. They were doomed.

However, fighting for their lives, the two frogs ignored the others and started jumping to get out of the pit.

The frogs at the top continued to tell the frogs in the pit to give up, as there was no way they would be able to jump out.

After jumping as high as they could over and over, one of the frogs listened to the others and gave up. He accepted the fate of his death. However, the other frog continued to jump with all of his might. The crowd of frogs yelled down the pit for the frog to just stop. He wouldn't make it.

However. the frog jumped even harder and persisted until he finally got out. Upon reaching the top, the other frogs said, "We thought there was no way any frog could jump that high, couldn't you hear us?"

The frog then signaled to the others that he was deaf, and he thought that the frogs standing around the pit were encouraging him the whole time.

The lesson of this story is that when it comes to your weight-loss success, the words of others can greatly impact your attitude and actions. Ignore the naysayers. Only engage with those who encourage and believe in your ability to succeed. Think about what you say to people before speaking so you can make sure what you're saying is supportive. Your support (or lack thereof) could make the difference between success and failure. Neila Rey, Founder of DAREBEE Fitness Resource and author of *100 No-Equipment Workouts,* summed it up best when she said, "I already know what giving up feels like. I want to see what happens if I don't."

Crabs in a Bucket

Are your friends hindering your weight-loss progress?

The story goes that if you put a single crab in a bucket, it can claw its way up and escape. However, if you put several crabs in a bucket, none will escape because as one attempts to climb out, the others will pull it back into the bucket. Simply stated, "crabs in a bucket" is a metaphoric phrase attributing a person or people stopping each other from bettering themselves, often pulling themselves down at the same time.

The phrase "*If I can't have it, neither can you*" best describes the "crabs in a bucket" mentality. When people with crab mentality see others around them succeeding in shedding weight, they subconsciously (or even consciously) attempt **to hold them back**.

For example, you are attempting to lose weight. However, your friend or friends persuade you that you look "fine" and that it's all right to indulge. This may come in the form of peer pressure to eat some of that birthday cake in the office, have the cookies, have the scoop of ice cream, or discouragement of going to the gym. The common phrase "*misery loves company*" is very true and can be seen in these types of situations.

What this means for you is your friends, co-workers, colleagues, or relatives will do what they can to hinder your weight-loss progress, or even stop you from simply attempting to succeed. Don't let them.

Did you know, the word "Diet" is derived from the Greek word *diaita* meaning "A way of living?" Food used to be consumed as fuel for the body. Today, however, it's used for comfort, to deal with stress, and enjoyment.

Here's some more good news. You don't have to worry about losing all the unwanted and unhealthy weight at one time. After all, you didn't gain all your weight at one time. And it is not a race to see who can lose the weight the fastest. In fact, many people who lose weight too quickly gain much, if not all of it, back. Some gain even more.

You just needed to lose a little bit at a time. You can reach a healthy weight that is easy to maintain by choosing to reduce your weight one ounce and one pound at a time.

That's the power of little, seemingly inconsequential improvements to your daily eating habits. It's the smallest changes to your eating habits and lifestyle done consistently over a long time (more than 66 days) that can make the biggest difference to achieve a healthy weight and, more importantly, keep it off. Researchers have found that it takes, on average, 66 days to form a new habit. What is important to remember is that old negative habits are difficult to break, and new positive habits are challenging to form and keep.

Darren Hardy described weight loss in his book, *The Compound Effect.* He talks about three buddies who grew up together. They all lived in the same neighborhood. They're all married and have average health and body weight. Friend one, called Larry, plods along doing what he's always done. He's happy, or so he thinks, but complains occasionally and nothing much ever changes.

Friend two, Scott, starts making small, seemingly inconsequential, positive changes. He begins reading 10 pages of a good book each day, cuts 125 calories from his diet, drinks pure water instead of soda. He also starts walking about a mile each day. Easy stuff anyone can do.

Friend three, Brad, makes a few poor choices. He buys a big screen TV and watches more programs. He watches the Food Channel and tries out new recipes, cheesy casseroles, and desserts. He also installs a bar in his home and adds one more alcoholic beverage per week.

At the end of five months, no perceivable differences exist between the three friends. No noticeable differences at the end of 12 months. But, at the end of 18 months, measurable differences start showing up. Within 25 months (a little over two years) you can see big differences between the three.

Scott has lost 33 pounds. Brad has gained 34 pounds; Brad weighs 67 pounds more than Scott.

There are other more significant differences.

Scott is doing very well at work, received a promotion, and his marriage is thriving. Brad's unhappy at work, his marriage is on the rocks, and he is miserable.

Larry is pretty much exactly where he was two years earlier.

Would you like to be 20, 30, 40, or more pounds lighter by this time next year?

Keep in mind, if you shed just one-half pound each week, you'll have lost 26 pounds in a year. Another way to think about it is if you lose just three pounds a month, in a year you will have dropped 36 pounds. I believe that you can lose two to three pounds per month. Would you agree with me that's certainly doable? Of course, it is.

THE THIRD PRINCIPLE FOR HEALTHY WEIGHT LOSS

The third principle as it pertains to weight loss is to eat organic, holistic/ whole foods, mostly plants.

In today's fast-paced, high-demand world, our culture has focused on convenience, and that includes how we eat. When we are hungry, it's much easier to go to the drive-thru, open a can, unwrap a package or pop a lid than it is to prepare a fresh meal. But according to holistic nutritionists, the cost of convenience has a dramatic impact on your health. With the epidemic rise of obesity and diabetes, the link to your health and what you eat has taken center stage. Many of you might be looking for a way not only to feed your bodies but heal yourself as well.

What are holistic foods? Holistic food is eating healthy food as close to its natural state as possible for optimum health and well-being. Hallmarks of holistic foods include unrefined, unprocessed, organic, and locally grown whole foods. Holistic or whole foods are foods that have been grown and nourished from the earth rather than manufactured and sold in a package. The contrast between these two kinds of foods lies in the difference in nutrient content. Fruits, vegetables, legumes, beans, nuts, seeds, and whole grains are a rich source of the vitamins and minerals that our bodies require.

Although processed foods may be enriched or enhanced with vitamins and minerals, they are rarely in the forms most bioavailable to our bodies. When you eat food that is vibrant and alive, you invite that vitality into your own body.

By choosing to eat more whole or holistic foods, you may experience health benefits, such as:

- Weight loss
- Increased energy levels
- Improved mood
- Better sleep
- Improved skin tone and texture
- Strengthened immune system
- Balanced blood sugar levels
- Reduced cholesterol and blood pressure levels
- Improved digestion and relief from constipation

Additionally, you may lower your risk for chronic illnesses that can be prevented or improved through diet, such as:

- Type 2 diabetes
- Arthritis
- Heart disease
- High blood pressure
- Cancer
- Colitis
- Gout

Eating whole, raw food is the simplest form to provide your body with proper nourishment. For a healthy snack, eat an apple, banana, carrot, celery, grapes, melon, avocado, or your favorite fruit or vegetable the way nature intended – raw and unprocessed. Another thing you can do is eliminate white flour or white rice because the white varieties are stripped of most of their nutrition and fiber. Other suggestions to eat whole foods and accomplish an eating behavior improvement and change:

- Eat cherries and nuts (unsalted/raw) as a snack

- Eat green leafy vegetables for salad and avoid high fat/high caloric salad dressings
- Eat berries (strawberries, blueberries, raspberries, blackberries, etc.) fresh or frozen
- Eat an orange instead of drinking a glass of orange juice
- Avoid fried foods

Unfortunately, most of us have a SAD food intake. SAD, which stands for Standard American Diet, is the primary cause of chronic disease and illness. But no matter how much proof or evidence exists on the health benefits of eating a mostly plant-based diet, the fact remains that most Americans will never give up their processed foods and SAD, fast food, lifestyle.

7

WHAT ARE YOU WAITNG FOR?

"There is more than one path to losing weight.
Make sure you are on the right path for you."

– David Medansky
The Overweight Person's Best Friend

A Dog Story

Based on a story told by Darren Hardy on *Darren Daily.*
Darren Hardy tells the story about a man, who one day was walking to work. As he walked, he noticed three dogs sitting on the front porch of an old farmhouse.

Two of the dogs got up and barked as the man passed by. However, the third dog did not bark. It was whining, moaning, and whimpering.

The man was curious as to why this one dog was not barking like the others. Unable to figure it out, he kept walking.

The next day, the man decided to walk to work again. Again, he noticed the three dogs sitting on the front porch of the farmhouse. And, again, two of the three dogs got up and barked while the third dog sat whimpering, moaning, and whining.

The man walked past the farmhouse for the entire week. Every day the same dog was on the porch moaning and groaning while the other two barked at him. Finally, frustrated with wondering why this dog was whimpering so much, his curiosity and concern got the better of him.

He had to find out what was wrong with this dog. Have you ever been so curious about something that you had to find out about it? Maybe how something was made, or how someone accomplished something special and unique?

He crossed the porch and knocked on the front door of the farmhouse. The farmer opened the door and asked, "How may I help you?"

The man asked, "Sir, is this your dog?"

"Yes," replied the farmer.

The man asked, "Well what's wrong with him? All week he's been sitting there moaning and groaning. The other two dogs bark at me, while he sits there."

The farmer replied, "Oh, well, he's sitting on a nail."

"What? Your dog is sitting on a nail? Why doesn't he just get off it?" the man asked.

The farmer smiled and responded, "Well, it doesn't hurt him enough."

Are you the dog sitting on the nail with being overweight? Are you tolerating being overweight?

Sometimes in life the pain we know is more comfortable than the pain we don't know. Especially with being overweight because of the increased risk for Type 2 diabetes, heart attack, stroke, and other health issues.

A lot of people tolerate being overweight because it doesn't hurt enough to do something about it. Do you justify and make excuses for being overweight? What needs to happen for you to do something about it?

To achieve healthy, sustainable weight loss, you will have to do something you don't want to do, something that will take effort and time. And you will constantly be pushed against the walls of your comfort zone. This is not a diet. Diets tend to be temporary, trendy, and hard to stick with. It's about living a healthy lifestyle.

The analogy of losing weight is similar to running a sprint versus running a marathon. A diet is a sprint. It has a finish line. Ninety percent (90%) of people who lose weight by dieting regain it. However, those who improve their lifestyle and eating habits keep the weight off because it's like running a marathon without a finish line. You just keep going.

The Top 10 Excuses Used to Delay Reducing Weight

1. I'll start after our vacation
2. I'll start after the holidays
3. Now's not the right time for me
4. I'm too busy
5. I'll start on Monday
6. It's too expensive. Healthy food costs too much
7. I'll start after our company picnic or party
8. I don't have time to follow a regimen
9. Many people who lose weight gain it all back so why bother?
10. I'm always hungry and cranky on a diet

In the movie *Rocky II*, Rocky Balboa's wife, Adrian (Talia Shire), wakes up from a coma and tells Rocky (Sylvester Stallone), "Win." Upon hearing Adrian tell Rocky to "Win," Rocky's manager, Mickey, (Burgess Meredith), says, "What are we waiting for?" The question posed to you is if you're wanting or needing to lose weight, "What are you waiting for?" Because if you're not going to start now, when will you start?

The biggest regret people have about losing weight is not starting a year earlier.

The second biggest regret about attaining a healthy weight is not starting now.

With respect to weight reduction, there are three types of people: 1) those who think about losing weight but do nothing, 2) those who talk endlessly about losing weight but do nothing, and 3) those who act to reduce weight. Which one are you?

There is never a perfect or right time to begin shedding your unwanted and unhealthy weight because tomorrow never comes. Have you used the excuse to justify delaying your weight-loss journey saying, "I'll start on Monday?" Or "I'll start after the holidays?" "After our vacation?" You get the idea.

Ask yourself this, "If I delay and put off until tomorrow what I can start today, what might happen?" Here's a hint to your answer. Tomorrow never comes until it is too late. It means if you keep putting off until tomorrow what you can start today, right now, right here, you will never start.

- What will happen if you don't improve and change your eating habits?
- Will you be like so many others and be diagnosed with Type 2 diabetes?
- Will you suffer a stroke or heart attack?
- Or will you end up in the hospital with some other debilitating disease or illness?

What is important for you to know is a study presented at the Society of General Internal Medicine 2017 Annual Meeting found that obesity has caused up to 47 percent more life-years lost than tobacco. The lead author of the study, Glen Taksler, PhD., investigated the underlying cause of a patient's death to understand the contributing factors. Dr. Taksler said, "The reality is, while we may know the proximate cause of a patient's death, for example, breast cancer or heart attack, we don't always know the contributing factor(s), such as tobacco use, obesity, alcohol, and family history." The study examined each major cause of death. They identified a root cause to understand whether there was a way a person could have lived longer. The conclusion: being overweight now causes more deaths than smoking.

Think about that. Obesity now causes more deaths than smoking. And seven out of every ten U.S. adults are overweight and four of those ten are clinically obese. Sobering statistics.

Researchers found that one in five deaths worldwide is linked to unhealthy eating habits. What you eat, and don't eat, may pose a bigger threat to your health than smoking, drinking, and other common risk factors for premature death.

Hippocrates, the Father of Medicine, said, "Just as food causes disease, it can be the most powerful cure." And, Heather Morgan, MS, NLC, summed up food for our bodies succinctly when she said, "Every time you eat or drink you are either feeding disease or fighting it." Which are you doing?

An extensive new study on diet trends around the globe ties poor eating habits to 11 million deaths around the world in 2017. The research, published in April 2019 in the journal, *The Lancet*, reported that bad eating habits was the primary factor that contributed to deaths linked to heart disease, Type 2 diabetes, and cancer.

Seventy percent of Americans (seven out of every ten) who are in the hospital are there because of their dietary habits and lifestyles. The sad part, much of it is preventable.

A 2009 study published in *The American Journal of Medicine* found that almost two-thirds of bankruptcies in the United States had a medical cause.

If you think it's expensive to eat healthy, you'd be wrong. Think of the costs for poor eating habits. It's expensive to get sick. The average out-of-pocket cost (after the insurance pays) per hospital stay after a heart attack is about $20,000.

Why wait until you get a disease or medical condition that puts you in the hospital when you can significantly reduce the risk and possibly prevent it simply by reducing weight? And, if you shed those unwanted and extra pounds, you'll feel better, have more energy, and probably want to be more active.

Here's another sobering fact: 80 percent (that's 8 out of 10) men and women over age 50 are pre-diabetic or diabetic. Diabetes is the sixth leading cause of death for men and women. Over a third of people with diabetes do not know they have it. That's why diabetes is sometimes referred to as the "silent killer." Being overweight is the number one factor increasing your risk for developing Type 2 diabetes. Type 2 diabetes is often a lifestyle disease, and it's preventable.

According to the Center for Disease Control and Prevention, "A person with diabetes is at high risk of heart disease, stroke, and other serious complications, such as kidney failure, blindness, and amputation of a toe, foot, or leg. In the last 20 years, the number of adults diagnosed with diabetes has more than tripled as the U.S. population has aged and become more overweight."

Maybe this statistic will scare you into taking action. Every year more than one million diabetics worldwide have a limb (foot, leg, hand, or arm) amputated because they did not and would not make the dietary improvements and changes that could reverse their condition.

If I am unable to inspire you to reduce weight in a healthy and sustainable manner, maybe I can use the fear of you being at higher risk for serious illness, infection, sickness, and possible death from your poor food choices and eating habits to motivate you. Perhaps you are not concerned about yourself. If not, then think of the impact that you contracting a preventable food-related illness could have on your family, your business, loved ones, and others.

Les Brown said, *"The graveyard is the richest place on earth, because it is here that you will find all the hopes and dreams that were never fulfilled, the books that were never written, the songs that were never sung, the inventions that were never shared, the cures that were never discovered, all because someone was too afraid to take the first step, keep with the problem, or determined to carry out their dream."*

Imagine your hopes and dreams being cut short because you failed to take care of yourself by simply reducing weight and making better food choices. It would be very sad if you had a heart attack or stroke, or a chronic illness that prevented you from accomplishing your potential. All of which could have been avoided by making a lifestyle change.

So, what will scare you enough to change your eating habits to lose weight and improve your health?

Perhaps you should go talk to people with Type 2 diabetes, people who have suffered a stroke or heart attack. Better yet, go talk to the loved ones who have lost parents, friends, relatives, and siblings way too early because of the poor food choices they made.

> *"On a regular basis I go over in my mind some of the most troublesome things I see about how people approach eating, and the wonder mess we have made out of a very simple thing."*
>
> **- Gabrielle ("Gabby") Reece,**
> Volleyball legend, *New York Times* best-selling author, and Nike's first female spokeswoman

I know from personal experience how fear can motivate. As you will recall, in July 2016 my doctor told me based on my lab results and being significantly overweight, I had a 95 percent chance for a heart attack. He gave me two options: 1) lose weight or 2) find a new doctor because he did not want me dying on his watch. With that sword hanging over my head, I shed 50 pounds (25 percent of my total body weight) during the next four months.

Unfortunately, many of my friends have not been so fortunate. They have either been diagnosed with Type 2 diabetes or have suffered a heart attack or stroke. I am blessed to have been lucky to avoid any of those ailments.

Do you need to end up in the hospital to modify your eating habits to lose weight and improve your health?

8

WEDDING CAKE, CHEESEBURGERS, AND WINE

"You must learn a new way to think before you master a new way to eat."

– Karen Salmansohn,
Multi-best-selling author and award-winning designer

There is a secret to achieving a healthy weight and lifestyle without needing willpower. The answer is one word. That one word is "No."

The only way to win against your willpower, self-control, and discipline for reducing weight is not to play. When you choose not to play, you win by default. This is what I mean. If you're attempting to reduce weight, willpower, self-control, and discipline, you will fail 100 percent of the time. When confronted with certain situations on your weight-loss journey, you need rules.

In this day and age, to reduce weight in a healthy and sustainable manner you need insane focus to counteract the onslaught of the crazy distractions and temptations working against you. These factions and factors include TV ads for food and restaurants, other people in your life, social occasions, special events, and holidays. You must be focused and create sacred boundaries – rules.

Special thanks to Darren Hardy who provided the analogy of choices we make as it relates to rules and winning without willpower, self-control, or discipline when confronted with having a cheeseburger, wine, and wedding cake.

Let's say you're at a friend's home for an outdoor barbeque. Your friend is making the most delicious cheeseburgers with a special cheese. The buns are fresh baked, not the store-bought type. And he will be serving your cheeseburger with all your favorite condiments. However, you're on a restricted diet to lose weight. What do you do?

Most people will succumb to the temptation to indulge in this special treat. Will you?

No, you won't because you're a vegetarian. You **don't** eat meat. Your decision is made for you. You **don't** have a choice.

Okay, you're at the same get-together and your friend being the gracious host that he is, offers you a glass of an expensive wine. In fact, it's your favorite wine. What do you do?

Do you accept the gesture and drink the glass of wine?

No, you won't because you're three months pregnant. Most women know they are not supposed to drink alcoholic beverages during their pregnancy. Again, your decision is made. You **don't** have a choice because you **don't** drink. You respectfully decline. The decision is easy.

Here is another example. You're attending a wedding. The wedding cake is spectacular. It was prepared by a world-renowned pastry chef. People's mouths are watering because it tastes as awesome as it looks. You, however, are watching your food intake because your mission is to lose weight. What do you do?

Most people will take a bite or two of the cake just for a taste.

You, however, graciously decline to partake because you're deathly allergic to nuts. The wedding cake has nuts. Your choice is made for you because you **don't** eat anything with nuts. If you do, you'll have a severe allergic reaction that can cause death.

These examples are to prove two things to you about rules:

1. you can resist when you ***must***, and
2. the only way to resist is if you ***must***.

Rules: A rule makes behavior decisions easy. Darren Hardy teaches: don't say you "can't" do something. Turn a "***can't***" into a "***don't***." Change saying, "I can't have a glass of wine," "I can't have a piece of cake," "I can't eat the cheeseburger" to "I don't eat beef" "I don't drink" and "I don't eat wedding cake." The reason, according to Darren Hardy, is that "can't" can be negotiated with. Instead, say you don't. "I don't drink," "I don't eat sweets on my diet," or, "I don't eat cheeseburgers while reducing weight."

'Don't' indicates to the one talking that you're in control. And, to yourself, that you're in control. 'Don't' indicates your statement is absolute.

'Can't' means you're not in control and that you can be convinced to indulge. Do not dismiss this because you think rules are too rigid. You follow rules all the time. You stop at red lights, you pay your taxes, you don't litter, etc. That's why establishing your own rules about eating will make it easier for you to succeed.

Systemize your own knowledge and create a set of eating rules for yourself. For example, you **don't** eat past 7:00 p.m. (or three hours before you go to sleep), you **don't** drink soda, diet soda, or fruit juices, because you only drink pure water, or whatever.

Would you like to eliminate refined sugars, bread, muffins, cake, and 90 percent of the Standard American Diet (SAD) and never waffle or waiver? Whatever situation you find yourself in won't matter. Be it birthday parties, holidays, special occasions, company functions, social gatherings, there is an absolute rule. That rule is under no circumstances will you answer anything but "No" or "No thank you," when offered something you know you shouldn't eat.

Just don't give in. Don't do it. Treat it like a pregnant woman does alcohol. For a pregnant woman, when offered alcohol, the answer should always be, "No." Or take someone who has an allergy to food such as nuts. When asked if they will make an exception to eating a few nuts or products made with nuts, the answer for them is always, "No." No matter what. Think of TINA.

You might be wondering… who is Tina? Tina is an acronym for the phrase, ***"There is no alternative."*** Think of TINA ("there is no alternative") when making your decisions pertaining to the food you consume. What is important to remember is beware of making exceptions because they tend to become the rule.

Make the choice once. If you make the choice once not to indulge in eating refined sugar, processed food, cake, pie, doughnuts, ice cream, sweets, bread, snacks such as chips, crackers, or pretzels, then you never need to make it again. You'll reduce a thousand choices into one. The choice not to eat chips, pretzels, cookies, sweets, processed foods, etc. is yours because of the rule that you don't eat these things.

You'll avoid all those situational, conditional, well/but circumstances that collapse on you every time to challenge (and win over) your willpower, discipline, and self-control. You've already made the decision and the answer will be, "No, I don't indulge or partake eating..."

You eliminate the need to make a choice because the choice has already been made. It's a hard and fast rule of absolutely, "No." No if's, but's, or exceptions, and no need to re-think the decision every time in every circumstance and situation.

Steve Jobs, co-founder of Apple, Inc. said, "Focusing is about saying no." This can and should be your own mantra for wanting to lose weight. Saying "No" to convenience foods, i.e., frozen microwaveable meals, going through the drive-thru for fast foods, ordering pizza, or picking up a bucket of fried chicken.

THE FOURTH PRINCIPLE FOR HEALTHY WEIGHT LOSS

The fourth principle for healthy weight loss is to eat slowly.

There's value to eating slowly. *Learning to eat slower is one of the simplest yet most powerful things you can do to improve your overall health.* We're all rushed, distracted, and too busy. Most people in the United States eat fast. Really fast. Rarely do people take the time to savor their food – or sometimes even to chew it properly.

Eating slower allows your body time to recognize that you're full. It takes about 20 minutes from the time you start to ingest your meal for the brain to signal you that you're satisfied. Most meals don't even last that long. As we learned from the Bliss Point, our food is scientifically engineered so that our brain never gets the signal to stop eating.

Eating slowly helps you feel satisfied before overeating. Imagine the extra calories, sugars, carbs, and fats you could eliminate simply by eating slower. Marc David, author of *The Slow Down Diet,* suggests if you eat breakfast in five minutes, increase the time to 10. If you normally take 10 minutes, increase it to 15 or 20. Give yourself a minimum of 30 minutes (half-an-hour) for lunch and dinner.

The benefits of eating your food slower include better digestion, better hydration, easier weight loss or maintenance, and greater satisfaction with our meals. Meanwhile, eating quickly leads to poor digestion, increased weight gain, and lower satisfaction. The message is clear: Slow down your eating and enjoy improved health and well-being.

Shoveling down your food means that you can sneak in a lot of extra calories before your stomach realizes what is going on. At the University of Rhode Island, researchers examined how eating speed affected the early stages of digestive processing by observing 60 young adults eat a meal.

What they found is:

- Slow eaters consumed 2 ounces of food per minute.
- Medium-speed eaters consumed 2.5 ounces of food per minute.
- Fast eaters consumed 3.1 ounces per minute. They also took larger bites and chewed less before swallowing.

In another University of Rhode Island study, researchers served lunch on two different occasions to 30 normal-weight women. When the researchers compared the difference in food consumption between the quickly eaten lunch and the slowly eaten lunch, here is what they found:

- When eating quickly, the women consumed 646 calories in 9 minutes.
- When eating slowly, the women consumed 579 calories in 29 minutes.

That is 67 *fewer* calories in 20 *more* minutes! For one meal.

If you extrapolate that to three meals per day, you can see how quickly those extra calories could add up. And here's another interesting twist: When the women ate their lunch quickly, they reported more hunger an hour later than those who ate their lunch slowly. So not only did eating quickly lead to greater food consumption, it also satisfied the women *less*.

Conversely, of course, eating slower meant less food yet longer-lasting satisfaction. Who knew?

Here are a few suggestions to help you slow down your eating behavior:

- Put the fork or spoon down between each bite.
- Avoid eating while driving.
- Avoid eating while working or at your desk.
- Avoid eating while watching television.
- Focus on eating and enjoying your food.
- Avoid distractions while eating. This can cause "mindless eating."

Mindless eating occurs when you are not aware that you just consumed an entire pint of ice cream or devoured a full bag of potato chips or other snacks because you weren't paying attention to the food you were stuffing into your mouth while focusing on other things.

As best you can, enroll your family, co-workers, and boss in creating more time and relaxation with meals. Find a "slow down" buddy to share meals and encourage each other to slow down while eating.

Eat only in a sitting position. Choose not to answer your cell phone, home phone, or texts while you're eating your food. When you slow down, savor a meal, pay attention to tastes and textures, and appreciate each mindful bite. This one small adjustment to your current eating routine can help you lose weight.

That reminds me of a story of when I ate fast. When I was in high school, my twin brother Larry, our friend Warren, and I sat down for lunch. My mon had just served Warren and Larry their food. My brother asked, "Aren't you going to give David his food?"

To which my mother responded, "I did. He ate it already."

Although we all sat down together to eat, I had cleaned my plate before Warren and Larry had a chance to get their food. It wasn't like I ate my food so much as I inhaled it.

May I share another example?

Great.

During my first year in college, about twice a week, a group of us played cards and ordered in pizza. Soon after we had a routine of playing, my roommate and friends suspected something wasn't quite right. One evening, after all the pizza had been eaten, Paul said, "I had only one slice, where's the rest?" Eric also said, "Hey, I only had one slice."

Jim looked at them and said, "Don't look at me, I only had one."

Jay shook his head, looked at me and asked, "David how many slices did you eat?"

Sheepishly, I replied, "I guess I had the rest." It was about five slices of an extra-large pizza.

After that, they limited me to two slices.

During my sophomore year, while dining in the cafeteria, I had six plates of spaghetti within 10 minutes. The girl serving the food in the cafeteria asked me on the sixth serving, "Are you eating this or dumping it?"

"I'm eating it," I responded.

She just shook her head.

About 20 minutes later I ran three miles. Surprisingly, I kept the food down.

A fraternity brother pinned the nickname Turbo on me because, as he put it, I ate so fast, I acted like a turbocharged engine guzzling gas.

Despite my poor eating habits, I weighed 155 pounds. I got away with eating a lot of food quickly because I exercised regularly. Can you relate to this?

While in college, I went to a restaurant to celebrate a friend's birthday. I ordered lobster tail. To my friends' amazement, I finished my meal last. They asked me if I was sick or felt ill. I said, "No, I wanted to enjoy it."

The point of this story is that I had the ability to eat leisurely, however, I chose not to do so at all other times. If you make a conscious decision, you can eat slower. Yes, you can adapt and modify your eating behaviors. I'm a perfect example.

9

THE "WINNER EFFECT"

"If you think in negative terms, you will get negative results.
If you think in positive terms, you will achieve positive results."

– Dr. Norman Vincent Peale,
American minister and author who is best known for his best-selling book, *The Power of Positive Thinking*

The "winner effect" is a term used in biology to describe how an animal, including a human, that won a few fights against weaker opponents is much more likely to win later bouts against stronger contenders.

Studies showed that fish and birds, rodents, and race car drivers, all follow a similar pattern. Winners keep on winning, and losers keep losing, even after researchers control for talent, skill, and other factors known to influence a win.

For example, researchers studied a mouse fight. One mouse was drugged to make him perform slower. He was matched with another mouse of equal physical size. Of course, the non-doped up mouse won.

Next the researchers had the winning mouse fight another mouse that was his equal in physical size. This time neither mouse was doped up, so it was a straight up fair fight. The previous victor won again.

Even when put they put the victor mouse up against bigger more aggressive mice, the probability of the first winning mouse winning again increased significantly. The study showed that after a mouse won a bout, it invariably went on to win again and again. Loser mice, meanwhile, continued losing.

Famously, before an important game against a tough offense Vince Lombardi called a young quarterback to throw passes against the defense. This young quarterback wanted to impress the great Lombardi and threw one completed pass after another.

Lombardi, furious, stormed up to this young quarterback yelling, "Are you trying to destroy my defense? Start throwing interceptions, damn it!" Apparently, the exercise was not to showcase the quarterback. It was intended to build the confidence of his defense.

The "winner effect" has powerful psychological benefits. This can be used to build your confidence on your weight-loss journey. Set a few small reachable goals such as drinking more pure water every day and eliminate drinking soda, diet soda, fruit juice, and fruit-flavored beverages.

A small taste of victory will build your confidence and increase your desire to do more to improve your eating habits. Even shedding two or three pounds the first few weeks is a victory.

Visualize improving your eating behaviors and shedding a few pounds. Because your mind doesn't know the difference. All it knows is it is a winner. And that is what winners do – they win.

THE FIFTH PRINCIPLE FOR HEALTHY WEIGHT LOSS

The fifth principle for healthy weight loss is to eat smaller portions.

Did you know your food portions have been supersized without you knowing it? It's true. The average dinner plate in the 1900s was nine inches in diameter. Over the years, the plate sizes have been made larger. In 2000, the diameter of the average size dinner plate was 11 inches. Today, the diameter of the average size dinner plate is 12 inches. Yet, in Europe, the diameter of the average size dinner plate is still nine inches. Perhaps this is one of the reasons that the United States has a weight problem.

Restaurants are notorious for giving portions that are two or three times more than what we should be eating. In restaurants, the diameter of the average serving plate is 13 to 15 inches. What this means to you is you are consuming almost 75 percent more food than is necessary.

So, what can you do when the server brings you your food that is too much to eat at one sitting? Simply cut it in half and ask for a to-go box. Put one-half in the to-go box. This will help you from overeating. Plus, you'll save money. It's like getting two meals for the price of one.

So, what can you do to reduce your food portions at home? Use a salad plate instead of a dinner plate. If you put the exact amount of food on a salad plate as on a dinner plate, the food on the dinner plate will look like you're getting less, and the food on the salad plate will look like you're getting more. It's an optical illusion. It's known as the Delboeuf Illusion.

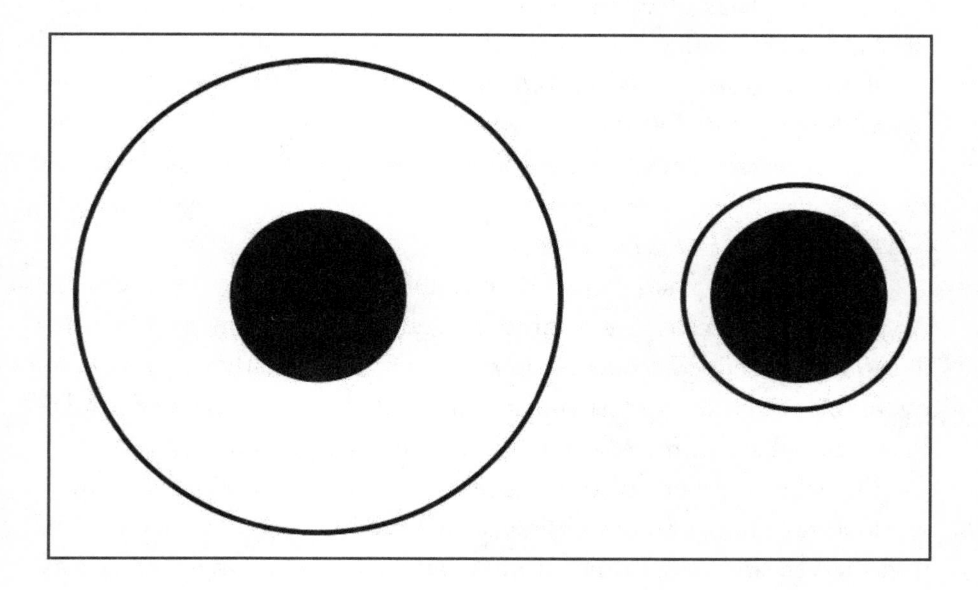

Franz Joseph Delboeuf, a Belgian mathematician and philosopher, first documented this phenomenon in 1865. Delboeuf started with two dots of equal size. He surrounded one dot with a large circle and the other dot with a small one. He noticed the second dot looked bigger.

Research suggests that choices, like how much to eat during a meal, are often made subconsciously. The problem arises because our brains are hardwired to mislead us in lots of little ways, which can have a big impact on our diets.

Brian Wansink and Koert Van Ittersum, professors of marketing at Georgia Institute of Technology, performed a series of experiments and tests to measure the effect of the Delboeuf illusion on serving behavior and perceptions of serving size. Their work appeared in the *Journal of Consumer Research.* Wansink and Van Ittersum found that a dinner plate size significantly impacts food consumption.

The professors asked Georgia Tech students to do various tasks of serving food. In one test, the students were to serve the same diameter (which represented the black dot in the center of the Delboeuf diagram) onto dinner plates of varying sizes, which represented the outer circles of Delboeuf's diagram.

What they found was the students served more food on the larger plates. They repeatedly under-served onto the smaller plates and over-served onto the larger ones. The students were unaware that they were doing this. The results demonstrated that the size of dinnerware you use to serve yourself on a day-to-day basis may significantly influence how much food you consume.

Van Ittersum said, "We are oftentimes our own worst enemy. And that's not because we want to overeat." Van Ittersum said that the illusion is embedded so deeply in our brains, it is nearly impossible to overcome. Even telling test subjects about it ahead of time, as they did in another phase of the research, didn't eliminate the bias.

Other researchers also measured serving behavior in the real-world atmosphere of a buffet line. They found the same results. People underserved and overestimated on small dishes, while the reverse was true for large dishes. People using the smallest dishes undershot the target serving by as much as 12 percent. However, people using the largest dishes took up to 13 percent more food than they intended.

A woman who had lost 125 pounds and kept it off told me that before she meets her friends at a restaurant, she looks at the menu. This gives her an opportunity to study the menu and decide before she goes to the restaurant what she would order. I told her that I did not need to look at a menu. That I could go to any restaurant and know what I would order. She asked me how.

As I explained to the woman, these are the magic words you can use when eating at a restaurant. Inform the server, "I am on a restricted diet. I'd like to order…a plain grilled chicken breast with a side of avocado," or "a grilled salmon with a side of steamed broccoli," or "a grilled steak (6 ounces or smaller) with a side of plain green beans/mixed green salad (with dressing on the side)," etc. Every time I've done this, the server has been more than willing to accommodate my request.

The beauty of this is that the server does not need to know why you are on a restricted diet. They do not know if you are attempting to lose weight, have food allergies, or any other reason. And none of the servers has ever asked me the reason.

What is important to remember is that it has been scientifically proven the size of your dinnerware affects your behavior for how much food you consume. Consider this: if you increase your caloric intake by just 50 calories per day because you're eating more than you should, you will gain an additional five pounds within one year. This is how the weight creeps up on us. It's gradual over a long period of time. Imagine reversing that trend and eating less simply by using a smaller plate. You'd most likely reduce your caloric intake by 50 calories per day. Which means that over time you'd get rid of extra weight.

As you will recall, if you shed just two pounds per month on average for 12 consecutive months, you'd weigh 24 pounds less within one year. The opposite holds true. This is why the size of your serving plate matters.

10

THE POWER OF WHY

"You can either have results or excuses. Not both."

– Arnold Schwarzenegger

There were two warring tribes that not so peacefully co-existed. One that lived in the lowlands the other high in the mountains. One day, the mountain people invaded the lowlanders, plundering and kidnapping a baby from the village.

They vanished with the child and took her back up to the mountains. The lowlanders, outraged at the disappearance of one of their own, were pushed into action.

The lowlanders, however, did not know how to climb the mountain. They did not know any of the trails that the mountain people used, or where to find the mountain people, or track them in the steep terrain.

Even so, they sent out their best party of fighters to climb the mountain and bring the baby home. The men attempted one method of climbing, then another, and another. They took one trail, then another, and then another. After several days of effort however, they had climbed only several hundred feet. Feeling hopeless and defeated, the lowlander men decided that the cause was lost, and they prepared to return to their village below.

As they were packing their gear for the descent, they saw the baby's mother walking toward them. They realized that she was coming down the mountain that they had not figured out how to climb. And then they saw she had the baby strapped to her back. How could that be?

One man greeted her and said, "We could not climb this mountain. How did you do it, when we, the strongest and most able men in the village, could not do it?"

The woman shrugged her shoulders and said intently, "It wasn't your baby."

Darren Hardy said, "The power of your why is what will power you to overcome any obstacle and achieve the seemingly impossible." What this means for you is if your "WHY" isn't big enough to shed weight, you won't.

"The Resistance"

You want to lose weight, right? I don't believe anyone wakes up in the morning wanting to be overweight and unhealthy. We all want to be healthy. So, what keeps you from losing weight? What blocks you at every turn? Stephen Pressfield in his book, *The War of Art,* called it, "The Resistance."

According to Darren Hardy, The Resistance has one sole mission – to keep things as they are. To keep you in your comfort zone. To prevent change. The Resistance will step in and immediately put a psychological chokehold on your ambitions to lose weight, become healthier, and prevent any forward progress of any kind. It will throw out a barrage of excuses for you to justify why you are unable to lose weight, i.e., "Hey, you are 'big boned." "You don't have the right genes." "You don't have time to eat healthy." "It costs too much." Does this sound familiar?

What this means for you is this is probably why you are among the 72 percent of U.S. adults who are overweight.

The Resistance is why people, like yourself, fail to lose weight and keep it off. It poses the greatest danger to your health and well-being. It is the reason many, like yourself, quit on your weight-loss journey. It is why you go back on your New Year's promise to lose weight every year.

So, how do you defeat The Resistance? You act. You defy The Resistance by taking action:

- You stop procrastinating.
- You stop thinking about it and start doing.
- You stop making excuses.
- You silence the voices of doubt.
- You decide to improve and elevate your daily eating habits.

HERE ARE FOUR FACTORS TO GET A HEALTHY WEIGHT:

Vision: What would life look like for you if you dropped 10, 20, 30, or more pounds? It is important for you to have a clear picture of how you will feel shedding the extra weight.

A Plan: You need a plan, a roadmap, a step-by-step process that will take you on your weight-loss journey. A well-charted map with a route – one that has been done by someone for you to follow that will help you achieve your weight-loss goals and improve your health.

A Mentor: A guide, someone who has already taken the trip, who has lost weight, and kept it off. Someone who is willing to take the time and energy to come back and lead you by the hand and escort you along your path toward your personal weight-loss goal.

Allies: Losing weight is tough. It is hard to do and often, it is lonely. When you are alone is when those little voices in your head do their best work on you. The Resistance shows up. The fog of temptation to indulge moves in. Your greatest asset will be an accountability partner.

This book will provide you with all the information you need to create your new and improved eating habits.

THE SIXTH PRINCIPLE FOR HEALTHY WEIGHT LOSS

The sixth principle for healthy weight loss is to get adequate sleep. Researchers have found that getting adequate sleep each night is a basic principle for maintaining good health and lowering your risk of gaining weight.

Why?

Because not getting the proper amount of sleep elevates your cortisol levels. Cortisol causes your body to go into fat storage mode. Elevated cortisol levels cause junk food cravings. And, not having enough sleep makes you tired, which increases your cravings for junk food. You'll know if you're tired all the time because you'll also be hungry all the time.

Getting adequate sleep is crucial for reducing weight. Getting enough sleep is required for turning off fat retention programs, reducing stress, reducing cortisol levels, and maintaining proper hormonal balance.

You need to get adequate sleep to successfully reduce weight. The average person who is sleep deprived will consume an extra 500 calories per day. It takes an average of reducing 500 calories per day for an entire week to lose one pound. Think about that. You're going in the wrong direction without adequate sleep.

It is better, for weight-loss purposes, to take a nap in the afternoon instead of exercising or working out. That is, you will lose more weight by taking a nap in mid-afternoon than you will if you work out. I know it sounds contradictory to what we've been taught; however, if you are sleep-deprived, it's better to take a nap. Nothing is more important than getting the proper amount of sleep when you're tired and when you're attempting to reduce weight.

Suggestions to accomplish behavior change for sleeping better at night:

- Turn your computer screens off an hour before bedtime
- Turn your television off an hour before bedtime
- Turn your Wi-Fi on your phone off at bedtime
- Put your phone on airplane mode
- Make the room as dark as possible
- Keep the room cool. Studies show that when a room is cool you sleep better

Another Frog Story

The story goes that if you put a frog in a pot of boiling water it will instantly leap out. However, if you put it in a pot filled with pleasantly tepid water and gradually heat it, the frog will remain in the water until it boils to death. The frog, supposedly, is unable to detect the gradual increase in temperature until it's too late.

This metaphor is often used in economics, business, and marketing to illustrate that change should be introduced gradually if it is to be successful. It also reveals an aspect of human psychology: we tend to accept things that creep up on us slowly and steadily. One day we wake up and find ourselves in boiling water. And such is the problem with our eating habits as it relates to our health.

The food industry is providing us with manufactured and processed foods. These edible products are scientifically engineered to be addicting. They are designed to optimize our cravings for sugar, salt, fat, and texture. And they are made to be convenient. Many people will go through a fast-food drive-thru, pick up a bucket of fried chicken, order a pizza, or pop a frozen meal in the microwave.

The chemicals used in manufacturing snacks, i.e., candy bars, protein bars, pretzels, chips, and other desserts are toxic. However, you won't notice how destructive they are to your body until it is too late. This is one reason more than 80 percent of people over the age of 50 are either a Type 2 diabetic or prediabetic. This is the reason for the increase in heart disease, stroke, and certain types of cancer. Keep in mind, nearly 70 percent of people in the hospital are there because of food related issues, primarily being overweight.

Are you the frog in the tepid water being slowly boiled until it is too late?

11

MINDLESS EATING

"Success is on the other side of your comfort zone."

– Orin Woodward,
New York Times best-selling author
and listed as a top leadership expert for Inc. Magazine

There is a story about a boy who once asked a wise old man what the secret to success is. After listening to the boy's question, the wise man told the boy to meet him at the river in the morning and he would be given the answer there.

In the morning, the wise man and the boy began walking toward the river. They continued on into the river, past the point of the water covering their nose and mouth. At this time, the wise man dunked the boy's head into the water.

As the boy struggled, the wise man continued to push him deeper into the water. After a few seconds, the man pulled the boy's head up so he could get air. The boy gasped as he inhaled a deep breath of air.

Once the boy had an opportunity to catch his breath and regain his composure, the wise man asked, 'What were you fighting for when you were underwater?"

The boy answered, "Air!"

The man said, "There you have the secret to success. When you want to gain success as much as you wanted air when you were underwater, you will obtain it. That's the only secret."

The lesson of this story is that success starts with the desire to achieve something. If your motivation is weak, your results will be weak as well. Think about your desire to lose weight and improve your health. How desperate are you to weigh less and be healthier? Don't allow your environment or other people to influence the things that you truly want. Just because other people are comfortable being overweight, out of shape, and in poor health doesn't mean you need to be too. What is important to remember is what Anne Wilson Schaef, American clinical psychologist and *New York Times* best-selling author, said: "Looking after my health today gives me a better hope for tomorrow."

THE SEVENTH PRINCIPLE FOR HEALTHY WEIGHT LOSS

The Seventh principle for healthy and sustainable weight loss is to focus on the food you eat by eliminating distractions that can cause "mindless" eating.

Does what's happening around you affect your eating? Some people tend to snack when watching TV. Others turn to food if other family members are eating, too. Where are you eating? At the kitchen table? In front of your computer? While watching TV? In your car driving? At your desk in your office or at work? A restaurant? Does where you eat increase the quantity you consume? If so, you might consider consciously changing the location of your meals.

According to a 2011 report from the U.S. Department of Agriculture, the average American spends two-and-a-half hours a day eating. However, more than half the time that we are eating, we are also doing something else. For instance, do you ever find yourself munching on a snack in front of the television and then next thing you know, you have eaten the entire bag? Were you even aware that you were consuming so much? This is "mindless" eating.

What is mindless eating? Mindless eating refers to an eating behavior where calories are consumed while the individual eating is unaware of the quantity being eaten or that he/she is eating in the first place. Mindless eating can occur any time that the brain is distracted, and the person is not aware of what or how much food he or she is consuming.

Mindless eating usually happens while another activity is simultaneously going on. Here are a few examples:

- Watching TV and eating chips out of a bag and before you know it half the bag is gone
- Sitting at work in front of the computer while the bowl of candy nearby slowly disappears, or the sandwich you were eating is gone
- Eating popcorn out of the bucket at the movies and munching away while you are engrossed by the film

Watching television detrimentally affects your eating habits, which can cause obesity. Studies show a direct correlation between watching television and weight gain. People tend to snack on calorie-dense processed foods while viewing the boob tube. Studies have shown that viewers consume 65 percent more calories from snacks while watching television.

According to Dr. Lilian Cheung, a nutritionist and lecturer at Harvard T.H. Chan School of Public Health, "mindless eating – a lack of awareness of the food we're consuming – may be contributing to the national obesity epidemic and other health issues."

There are several factors that contribute to mindless eating. Some of these are:

- **Boredom.** Eating when you're not hungry because you are bored and eating food or snacks is going to give you something to do.
- **Distracted eating.** You are eating when your mind is sidetracked by television, working, driving, watching a movie, or other diversions.
- **Awareness.** Overeating because you are unaware just how much food you are consuming because you are eating directly out of

the bag or box, or not measuring portion sizes. As an example, grabbing a few handfuls of nuts out of the can or jar. Each handful could have as many as 100 calories each.

- **Emotions.** Some individuals turn to food for comfort when they are sad, anxious, upset, hurt, or angry.
- **Commercials and advertisements.** An outside source, such as food advertisements or television commercials, may contribute to mindless eating.

Have you noticed that commercials displayed on the screen during prime time and late at night are prominently for food and restaurants? They're designed and created to entice you to eat more. Further, eating late at night is the worst time to chow down. To add insult to injury, the advertisements usually depict thin people. If you have a poor self-image, you might consume more food to comfort yourself. Television commercials provide conflicting, confusing, and misleading information about proper nutrition. Because of this, people who watch a lot of television tend to have a poorer understanding of health eating.

One study found 34 percent of viewers were more likely to order high-fat, high-sugar foods from menus than those who didn't watch television. Who wants to order a pizza from Pizza Hut, Little Caesars, or Domino's? Perhaps by keeping a food journal you'll discover you're watching a lot more television than you thought.

What can you do to combat a television eating habit?

Do a few push-ups between commercials. The average commercial break is two to five minutes. Instead of getting up to grab a snack, do some push-ups. Even if you start with five. You can build up to doing 25 to 50 push-ups during a commercial break. Do some leg lifts. Again, start slowly and build up. Before you know it, you'll be doing 25 to 50 leg lifts during each commercial break along with your push-ups.

Not fond of leg lifts? Do squats. Or grab light-weight dumbbells. There are many things you can do during a commercial break to get some physical activity. Imagine, you won't need to go to the gym to do a workout. You'll save time and money.

The average one-hour television show has between seven and 10 commercial breaks. If you can build up to doing just 25 push-ups during just four commercial interruptions, you'd have done 100 push-ups during the show. Do it gradually if you haven't done much or any exercise in a while.

You might consider tracking how many hours you spend watching television. It may surprise you how much time you're wasting in front of the screen. With Netflix and other subscription channels, there are no commercials. And during the COVID-19 pandemic, these subscription networks gained millions of new viewers. What this means for you is you need to be aware of how many hours you are sitting in front of the boob tube without moving.

Do you watch television in your bedroom? This can disrupt sleep and cause other health issues. Research shows that the nighttime glow streaming from the television throws off biorhythms, messes with hunger signals, and has a direct correlation to weight gain. A simple solution is to remove the culprit from the bedroom or make certain it has been off an hour before you go to sleep.

What else can you do to curtail mindless eating?

Pre-portioning out your servings. For example, instead of grabbing a handful of nuts, count out 10. Eat them slowly, one at a time, instead of putting the entire handful into your mouth. Avoid eating while watching television. If you do eat or snack while watching TV, don't eat out of the bag. Instead, portion out an individual serving into a small bowl.

Avoid eating your meals such as dinner or lunch while working at your desk or in front of your computer. Take at least 30 minutes to eat lunch and 30 minutes to eat dinner. Focus on the food you are consuming.

Avoid eating while driving. If you choose to go through the drive-thru at a fast-food place, park and eat your meal before driving to your destination.

Keep tabs on your eating behavior for a few weeks. Then look for patterns. If it appears there's a relationship between eating and feelings, think of ways to meet the emotional needs without turning to food. Ask people in the support community for suggestions. Or, if they will be an accountability buddy you can talk to so you avoid comfort eating. Maybe take a walk, do some yoga or quick exercise. Play with your dog or cat. Find other ways to deal with frustration.

So, the opposite of "mindless" eating is "mindful" eating. Mindful eating is a method that allows you to gain control over your eating habits. Controlling your eating habits has been shown to help with weight loss.

What is mindful eating?

Mindfulness is defined as a state of being conscious or aware of something. In other words, increasing your awareness of your physical, cognitive, and emotional state, as well as the environment and events you are experiencing at the present moment. To be a mindful eater means that you are fully aware of the food you are eating, how much you are consuming, and can really enjoy and savor the flavor of the food. Kati Konersman, RD, CDE, summed it up best stating, "Mindful eating is eating with attention while paying attention." What this means for you is mindful eating is eating with intention.

Some tips to become a mindful eater are:

- Slow down. Eat slower.
- Think about why you are eating. Is it because you are hungry or is it because you are bored? Maybe you are upset, anxious, or excited?
- As best as possible, eat your meals at a kitchen or dining room table.
- Avoid eating while watching TV or in front of your computer.
- Pay attention to what you are eating and how much you are eating.

According to Megrette Fletcher, M.Ed., RD, CDE, "Challenge yourself to notice the two parts of every food choice: What and how much."

12

ROUTINES, BEHAVIORS, AND HABITS

"Change your habits, change your life."

– Thomas C. Cooley

There is a story about a king who wanted to test his subjects to see how they would handle obstacles in their way. So, he had a giant boulder placed in the middle of one of the village's busiest streets. Then he hid nearby to see who, if anyone, would try to move the large stone out of the way.

First, some wealthy merchants walked by. They walked around the boulder, complaining that the king hasn't been maintaining the roads very well.

A short time later, more villagers came upon the boulder. A few commented about the boulder not being there before and wondered how it got there. They also walked around it. None of them made an effort to move the boulder.

Soon thereafter, a peasant walked by, heading home with his arms full of food for his family. When he came upon the boulder, he put his groceries down and attempted to move it out of everyone's way. Other people passing by ignored the peasant. None offered to help. It took him a while to move it, but he eventually succeeded.

After the peasant gathered up his groceries to carry on home, the king appeared. He handed the peasant a pouch filled with gold coins. The king explained that the bag of gold was a reward for the peasant because he had taken the time and energy to move the boulder out of the road for the convenience of others who would be travelling the road in the future.

The boulder in this story represents the obstacles and challenges you might face during your weight-loss journey. The peasant in this story was taught by the king that every obstacle and challenge you face offers an opportunity to improve. If you take the time and make the effort to push through the obstacles and challenges in front of you to improving your eating habits, you may end up being much better off simply by making the effort.

This story also offers a lesson of personal responsibility. The boulder represents your excess weight. Are you complaining about being overweight and blaming others while doing nothing, much like the wealthy merchants who blamed the king for the roads not being well-maintained? It is your responsibility to improve your eating habits to lose weight. No one else can do this for you.

Routines Become Behaviors, Behaviors Done Consistently Become Habits

Before we get into HOW to change and improve your daily eating routines, I'd like to offer you a daily ritual to start each day. It is optional. You only need to do it if you choose to do so. Read the words below, out loud, to start each new day.

I begin the day expecting amazing things.
I begin the day being grateful for what I have and what I will receive.
I begin the day open to receiving new ideas,
new information, and new connections.
I begin the day letting go of what's not serving me.

Some refer to this as "bless and release."
I begin the day being a positive influence on others.
"I am whole, perfect, strong, powerful, loving, harmonious, grateful, confident, healthy, and happy.
I am love. I am compassionate.
I am good fortune.
I am positive energy flowing to the higher good.

Napoleon Hill began his day reciting, "O Divine Providence, I ask not for more riches, [instead, I ask for] more wisdom with which to make wiser use of the riches you gave me at birth, consisting in the power to control and direct my own mind to whatever ends I desire."

It is the small, comfortable, daily steps toward change and improvement in your eating routine and habits that will give you weight-reduction success. You will not reduce your weight until you improve and change your eating behaviors. What is important to remember is that behaviors done consistently over a long time become new habits. A string of behaviors is a habit. Losing weight and being able to keep it off is not like getting a vaccination. You don't get one shot and forget about it. It doesn't work that way.

For a new behavior to happen consistently, you must find a way to remove all thinking, all discipline, and all willpower from the equation. If you need to rely on any of that, you're screwed. Have you experienced a lack of willpower or discipline? Yeah, if you're being honest, you have, as seen from all your past resolutions, diets, and failed promises.

Improving your eating behaviors to become new habits will eliminate your need for self-control and willpower. Brushing your teeth is a habit. You don't need self-control to brush your teeth; you do it without thinking. A habit requires no decision making because the decision has already been made. With your improved eating habits, you don't make decisions, you don't think, you just eat healthy because that is how you eat.

The approach you will learn in this lesson is based on the Keystone Habit discussed by Charles Duhigg in his book, *The Power of Habit*, whereby changing one key habit can change your entire life. A Keystone Habit is more important than others because it leads to the development of other habits. While Keystone Habits don't necessarily create a direct cause-and-effect relationship, they start a chain effect that produces other positive outcomes.

Charles Duhigg told the story how Paul O'Neill changed one Keystone Habit to transform the American Aluminum Company of America, also known as ALCOA, a corporation that manufactures everything from the foil that wraps Hershey's Kisses and the metal in Coca Cola cans to the bolts that hold satellites together, into an extremely profitable organization and a mainstay of safety.

According to Duhigg, after Paul O'Neill became the new CEO of ALCOA, he spoke with Wall Street investors and stock analysts on a blustery day in October 1987. A few minutes before noon, O'Neill took the stage and said, "I want to talk to you about worker safety. Every year, numerous ALCOA workers are injured so badly that they miss a day of work. I intend to make ALCOA the safest company in America. I intend to go for zero injuries."

The audience was confused. Usually, a new CEO talks about profit margins, new markets, and collaboration. But O'Neill said nothing about profits. He didn't mention any usual business buzzwords.

Eventually, a person in the audience asked about inventories in the aerospace division. Another asked about the company's capital ratio. O'Neill responded, "I'm not certain you heard me. If you want to understand how ALCOA is doing, you need to look at our workplace safety figures. Profits do not matter as much as safety."

When the presentation ended, the investors and analysts bolted out the doors. One investor dashed to the lobby to find the nearest pay phone. He called 20 of his largest clients and told them, "There's a crazy hippie in charge who is going to kill the company." He strongly suggested and advised them to sell ALCOA stock without delay.

Later, that same adviser admitted it was the worst piece of advice he gave in his entire career. Within a year of O'Neill's speech, ALCOA profits soared to a record high. By the time O'Neill left ALCOA in 2000 to become Treasury Secretary, ALCOA's annual net income was five times larger than before he arrived.

So how did O'Neill transform ALCOA, a large, dull, and dangerous company to work for, into an extremely profitable organization and one of the safest companies to work for? By attacking one area of interest, ALCOA's concern for safety – a Keystone Habit. That single change to improve safety rippled throughout the entire organization.

O'Neill said, "I knew I had to transform ALCOA. But you can't order people to change." This same concept applies to weight reduction. We all know what to do, we just don't do it. No one can order or command you to change your eating habits and behaviors. As to forcing people to comply with directions, O'Neill said, "That's not how the brain works. So, I decided I was going to start by focusing on one thing. If I could start disrupting the habits around one thing, it would spread throughout the entire company."

This can work for you in your personal life and weight-reduction journey. Just pick one Keystone Habit or one key behavior to change. Focus on improving one thing. It could be one aspect of the food or beverages you eat or drink or one behavior you do while eating a meal. Just pick one to start.

Darren Hardy provided the inspiration for this blueprint to change and improve your eating behaviors to achieve your weight reduction goals with weekly planning in his *Sunday Planning System.* He suggested not to get caught up into the complete makeover or the life renovation idea because it will end up being too much, triggering a collapse in discipline.

Hardy explained that radically making a change or going to an extreme will bring the entire weight-loss process down like a house of cards. Darren Hardy, like Charles Duhigg, trusts that if you disrupt the habit of doing one thing, it will spread throughout your entire lifestyle.

Each Sunday, plan your week. Plan your meals. Plan how you will handle certain situations that may pose a challenge or obstacle to sticking to your new eating habits.

Set the behavior you want to improve for the week. Focus on one or two behaviors to improve upon each week.

When you focus on changing and improving one key habit, you will notice it will have a ripple effect on your body, mind, and spirit, and positively affect almost every other aspect of your life. People fail to reduce weight in a healthy and sustainable manner because they lose focus, make exceptions, and get sidetracked. Each year, people make resolutions to lose weight. Eighty percent of those will fail within the first few weeks. They are not committed to reducing weight.

Commitment, according to Darren Hardy is defined as, *"Doing the thing you said you were going to do long after the mood you said it in has left you."*

13

HOW YOU DO ANYTHING IS HOW YOU DO EVERYTHING

"Do what is easy, and your life will be hard.
Do what is hard and your life will become easy.

– Les Brown,
World-renowned motivational speaker

One afternoon, a carpenter, who had been with the same company for more than 30 years, told his boss that he was ready to end his career and spend time with his wife and family. He would miss his work, however, he felt he needed to spend more time with the people who were important to him.

The owner of the company was saddened by this news, because this carpenter had been a good, reliable employee for many years. He asked the carpenter if he could do him a favor and build just one more house.

Reluctantly, and after a bit of persuasion from the owner, the carpenter agreed to build just one more home.

The carpenter's heart just wasn't in building this last home. He lost focus and dreamed of spending time with his family. Because he was not fully engaged in this project, his normal work ethic waned and his efforts were mediocre at best. He chose to use inexpensive and inferior materials. He cut corners wherever he could. The craftsmanship was shoddy. It was a poor way to finish such a dedicated career that he once had.

When the carpenter had finished, his boss came to inspect the house. He gave the key to the carpenter and said, "This house is my gift to you for all the hard work you have done for me over the years."

The carpenter was surprised and overwhelmed with his boss' generosity. He graciously accepted the gift. After his boss left, the carpenter sat for a moment to ponder his decision to put forth less than his best effort. Had he known the home was for him and his family, he would have made his usual effort to create a high-quality home.

The same idea applies to how you take care of your own body. Dr. Bob Martin, Certified Clinical Nutritionist (C.C.N.), host of "The Dr. Bob Martin Show," the largest syndicated alternative health show in the U.S., said, "If you wear out your body where are you going to live?"

Each and every day that you wake up you have an opportunity to do your best and be your best. Yet many of you often do mediocre work. Why? Shouldn't we strive to improve each day?

As we get older, we find ourselves shocked that our lives aren't what we had hoped they would be. The "house" (our bodies) we built to live in has a lot of flaws due to a lack of effort. Unfortunately, you are unable to go back and rebuild it in a day or two. It takes time to repair the damage done. There is a saying, "Life is a do-it-yourself project." And so is maintaining and taking care of your body. Your attitude and daily food choices help build the quality of life you will have in the future. Build carefully.

THE EIGHTH PRINCIPLE FOR HEALTHY WEIGHT LOSS

The eighth principle for healthy weight loss is to give your body 12 to 14 hours each day to digest and process the food you consume. This discussion is about intermittent fasting. Whenever fasting is mentioned, there is always the same eye-rolling response. Starvation. Can you relate to this? Did you roll your eyes, too?

Have you seen the ads and online messages about intermittent fasting? With all the hype about it, you may feel it's just another modern diet fad. The truth is fasting is thousands of years old.

Fasting is not starvation. Starvation is the *involuntary* absence of food. It is neither deliberate, nor controlled. Starving people have no idea when and where their next meal will come from.

Fasting, is the *voluntary* withholding of food for spiritual, health, or other reasons. The two terms, "starvation" and "fasting," should never be confused with each other. In a sense, fasting is part of everyday life. The term 'break-fast' is the meal that breaks the fast, which, for many people, is done daily.

Fasting is one of the most ancient and widespread healing traditions in the world. Hippocrates, who is widely considered the father of modern medicine, prescribed the practice of fasting and the consumption of apple cider vinegar as treatments. Hippocrates wrote, "To eat when you are sick, is to feed your illness."

Writer and historian Plutarch wrote, "Instead of using medicine, better fast today." Plato said, "I fast for greater physical and mental efficiency." Aristotle, his pupil, also fasted. According to Paracelsus, one of the three fathers of Western medicine, "Fasting is the greatest remedy – the physician within."

Fasting isn't abnormal. It's a natural healing process. Fasting is widespread. Fasting remains part of virtually every major religion in the world. Jesus Christ, Buddha, and the prophet Muhammed all shared a common belief in the power of fasting for cleansing or purification. In other words, healing.

The practice of fasting varies between cultures and religions. In Buddhism, food is often consumed only in the morning, and followers fast from noon until the next morning daily. In addition to this, there may be various water-only fasts for days or weeks on end. Greek Orthodox Christians may follow various fasts over 180-200 days of the year. Crete is considered the poster child of the healthy Mediterranean diet. Yet most of the population of Crete followed the Greek Orthodox tradition of fasting. Muslims fast from sunrise to sunset during the holy month of Ramadan.

It's only until recently in human history that people have not gone for extended periods of time without food. Throughout our evolutionary history, there would be periods lasting days, weeks, or months during which food resources were scarce.

Today, in our modern society, we are blessed, or cursed depending on the source, with an abundance of food. Unfortunately, much of our food today is manufactured or processed. We overconsume products full of sugar, dairy, and grains that are high in calories and unhealthy fats. Yet, with all this overconsumption, our bodies do not get enough nutrients.

Most people are overconsuming grain. When you eat too much grain, you overconsume Omega-6. Too much Omega-6 causes inflammation to your body. Dr. Lori Shemek wrote about this in her best-selling book, *FATflammation!* Grain is in virtually all processed foods. The Food Pyramid in the U.S. is a solid base of grain. Also, you're probably eating a lot of processed sugar made from grains – specifically corn – without realizing it. And this causes inflammation in your body.

Dr. Peter Osborne, the clinical director at the Origins Healthcare in Sugarland, Texas, and author of the best-selling book *No Grain, No Pain,* provides a great analogy. Dr. Osborne says to imagine that you go home from work every day and prepare your meals, eat, but never do your dishes. The dishes keep piling up in the sink. Eventually, they start spilling out of the sink and onto the countertop. Before you know it, you have bugs eating the debris of the food left on the dishes. And you have a huge mess in your house because you didn't do the dishes.

Dr. Osborne says that's what happens in your stomach. When you put too much in and don't have normal "housekeeping," the stomach becomes overwhelmed, and your gastrointestinal system becomes a breeding ground for bacteria. And when you eat all the time and don't give your stomach a rest, it becomes exhausted. Your gut needs a vacation!

This is where fasting comes in. You're giving your body a chance to clean the dishes, so to speak. It gives your body a chance to rest and repair itself.

My friend Dr. Rachel Smartt told me another analogy to explain the importance of fasting. Dr. Smartt described fasting as your body being a power lawn mower and the food you consume being wet grass. As you mow wet grass, it sticks to the undercarriage and begins to clog the mower's blade. To keep the mower's engine from overheating, you must clean the undercarriage and remove the wet grass. Otherwise, the accumulation of the wet grass will make the engine work harder and eventually cause it to burn out. This is what happens when you put too much food into your system. Fasting gives your body time to cleanse itself. If you don't allow your body time to clean itself, it will put a strain on your digestive system and other organs.

There are many types of fasts. For instance, there is intermittent fasting, a water fast, a bone broth fast, a green juice fast, a liquid nutrition fast, and a fasting mimicking diet, to mention just a few. Because this can become a very confusing topic, this discussion is limited to intermittent fasting.

There is a difference between intermittent fasting and extended fasting or long fasting. An extended fast or long fasting is more than 36 hours. If you decide to do an extended fast, it MUST be under the supervision of a medical doctor or qualified health professional. Please, do NOT do an extended fast without proper medical supervision.

What happens to your body when you fast?

When you fast intermittently, insulin levels go down and glucagon goes up, which has been shown to have benefits such as increased metabolism, more energy, improved mood, and weight loss.

Fasting can also increase the diversity of bacteria in your gut, which is important for your immune system and overall health. Researchers have linked daily fasting to activation of the gene that strengthens the gut barrier to protect us from harmful microbes, contaminants, and other substances that can trigger immune reactions.

How and when do you fast?

Intermittent fasting, also called "time restricted feeding," is the practice of eating food within a certain time period during the day. Intermittent fasts can last as little as four hours or as long as 36 hours. Anything longer than 36 hours is considered an extended fast and ***must*** be done under the supervision of a medical doctor or qualified health professional.

For those of you who've never done an intermittent fast, begin with one of the most common approaches to intermittent fasting: eat your meals within an eight-hour period and avoid food, except pure water, during the next 16 hours. Why 16 hours? Some research suggests that 16 hours is the optimal amount of time for creating the caloric restriction that happens during fasting and to give your cells time to cleanse themselves. However, other experts feel that 12 to 14 hours is sufficient to give your body time to cleanse itself. Make certain you drink between eight and 16 ounces of water when you first wake up. This will help reduce morning hunger and prolong the fast and improve the cleansing process.

"The best of all medicines is resting and fasting."

– Benjamin Franklin

This is what an intermittent fast could look like: You finish dinner at 7:00 p.m. and you don't eat again until 7:00 a.m. That's it! That is a 12-hour intermittent fast.

This is really the easiest way to start any kind of fasting. You might already be implementing this into your weight-reduction journey without realizing it.

Be realistic about intermittent fasting. There will be times when you're going out with friends for dinner or attending other events that might be outside your time frame for eating. If this happens don't worry about it. You don't need to make a religion out of intermittent fasting. It is not a hard and fast rule. You don't need to do intermittent fasting every day. These are just guidelines to shift your hunger habit.

Experts have their own views and opinions about what is the best way to do intermittent fasting, whether it is 12, 13, 16, or 18 hours. You need to figure out and determine what is best for you. If you work the night shift or wake up at different hours, make your own fasting schedule. The concept is that you're eating most of your food during a six- to eight-hour period and you're doing it when your body has adapted to the process. Go at your own pace. You don't want to force your body into an intermittent fasting regimen if it's not ready.

Here's another thought: Don't force yourself into eating during only a six- to eight-hour window of time if you're hungry the rest of the time. Intermittent fasting is not right for you at this moment. That doesn't mean you won't be able to do this in the future. Make small adjustments to your daily eating routine consistently over a long period of time until it becomes your habit.

Even though intermittent fasting has many benefits to help heal your body, it doesn't mean you can eat anything you want such as processed foods and junk food, and it doesn't mean you can eat as much as you want. You still need to eat whole (holistic) foods and watch your portion sizes. If you keep eating 2,000 calories a day or more, you're not going to shed those extra pounds. One caveat: if you're doing intensive exercise or heavy physical activity, you'll need to adjust your caloric intake to a higher amount to make sure you don't put your body into starvation mode.

Autophagy = 100 percent natural cellular detox

Are you familiar with the term autophagy? (Pronounced "aw-TOFF-uh-gee.") The most basic definition of autophagy is the body's self-cleaning process that removes damaged proteins, stored fat, and debris, other waste products inside cells. But unlike trendy "cleanses" and "detoxes," autophagy is 100 percent physiological. What is important to remember is it is a natural biological mechanism. Fasting advocates say autophagy allows your own biology to restore vitality, slow down the aging process, prevent disease, and help you bust through a weight-loss plateau.

What this means for you is this type of cleanse doesn't involve drinking any weird beverages, eating tasteless cardboard-like food, or torturing yourself with hours of excessive exercise. Autophagy is completely natural and happening inside of you all the time to different degrees, even when you don't realize it. It's as natural for our cells to self-cleanse (autophagy literally means self ["auto"] – eating ["phagy"]) as it is for them to undergo normal wear and tear.

Autophagy declines with age and poor diet. This can cause cells to be damaged faster. Research has shown that intermittent fasting or healthy caloric restriction can activate autophagy. Now you have a less-complicated anti-aging strategy that can increase cellular repair and renewal every day. That's the idea advanced by Japanese cell biologist Yoshinori Ohsumi, who won the Nobel Prize in Medicine in 2016 for his research on autophagy. Ohsumi proved autophagy to be the one true physiological detox program that is 100 percent backed by science.

Persistent myths about fasting – they're wrong

Let's take a minute and look at a couple of persistent myths about fasting. One is that fasting shuts down the thyroid gland in women. Thomas Delauer, a celebrity trainer and author of the book, *Top Ten Intermittent Fasting Hacks: Ten Key Tips to Make Fasting Easier & More Effective* said that is just misinformation. He doesn't know where that misinformation comes from.

The other myth about fasting is that it slows your metabolism and forces the body into starvation mode, causing the body to retain fat. A review of more than 30 independent studies demonstrates that the opposite is true. The studies indicate that intermittent fasting can accelerate and enhance weight loss. The studies found that intermittent fasters shed an average of seven to 11 pounds during a 10-week period.

Here's a summary of benefits of fasting gleaned from various books and articles on the topic:

- **It improves energy levels.** People who regularly practice intermittent fasting have noticed improved energy levels.

- **It reduces inflammation.** Numerous studies have shown that fasting reduces the number of inflammatory cytokines produced in your body.
- **It stimulates fat burning.**
- **It takes stress off your digestive system.** Digestion is a stressful and demanding process on the body. You can reduce the stress level of your digestive tract by fasting and allowing it to heal and repair itself.
- **It stimulates cellular autophagy.**
- **It improves genetic repair processes.** Research has shown that cells have a greater lifespan during times of famine and food scarcity. Fasting enhances the cellular rejuvenation by acting on certain genetic repair processes.
- **It can help improve insulin sensitivity.** Insulin, which is a hormone, helps your body burn sugar for fuel. Improved insulin sensitivity helps people with insulin resistance and Type 2 diabetes.
- **It can help reduce your risk for chronic disease.** All chronic diseases are caused by chronic inflammation. Fasting is the most powerful nutritional method to reduce inflammation in your body.

When you reduce your inflammatory levels, you influence your genes to induce better health for all your organs, systems, tissues, and the cells of your body. Doing this will greatly reduce your risk of chronic disease and acts as an anti-aging mechanism.

Most people shouldn't need to purchase products that claim to reduce inflammation if you are in the habit of intermittent fasting at least three times per week. **I don't mean medicine: Always consult with your medical doctor or qualified health professional before stopping any anti-inflammatory medication you are currently prescribed.**

It can help you improve your food choices. Many of you might be struggling with mindless eating and have struggled with sugar, carbs, dairy, and other cravings. Fasting can help you realize that these cravings are mental and emotional and that you can overcome them.

It can help improve your mood. Fasting elevates your ketone levels. When this happens, many people experience improvement in their mood, have higher mental clarity and creativity. Usually achieving this improvement requires an extended fast of three to four days.

The information on fasting is presented for educational purposes only and is not designed to treat or cure any health conditions. If you want to incorporate fasting strategies into your weight-loss journey, please consult with your medical doctor or qualified health practitioner first to make sure it is OK for your unique health situation and/or condition.

There are some people who should NOT fast. These include, but are not limited to, pregnant women, newborn babies, young children, high-level athletes who do intense training, individuals with a history of eating disorders, Type 1 diabetics, and individuals with pathological cachexia. (Cachexia is a condition that causes extreme weight loss and muscle wasting. It is a symptom of many chronic conditions, such as cancer, chronic renal failure, HIV, and multiple sclerosis.)

A Horse Story

A few years ago, while in Las Vegas, I met the owner of a "prized" thoroughbred racehorse. During our conversation, he explained to me how he made certain his horse got the best nutritional supplements and ate the healthiest food to optimize the horse's performance. He boasted how he hired the best licensed and certified veterinarian to thoroughly examine the horse each week. He bragged how the horse got the best dental care available.

The horse had his own personal trainer to exercise it every day. He made sure that the horse's environment was optimal for social interaction to keep the horse's spirits up. No expense was spared on maintaining the horse's health so the horse could perform at its best. Indeed, the man's knowledge about what the horse needed, and was provided, for optimal performance was remarkable.

However, what made the biggest impression on me meeting this owner was how he cared for himself. You see, this gentleman was at least 75 pounds overweight. When the waiter served the owner's lunch, it was a huge hamburger loaded with cheese, bacon, lettuce and tomato, ketchup, mustard, and mayo. Of course, there was a side of golden French fries and an ice-cold Coke to wash down the food. It was apparent and obvious that this owner was more concerned about the health and care of his racehorse than himself.

Pushing the conversation, I asked the owner how often he'd get a check-up from his doctor. The owner scoffed at the idea. His response, "I haven't been to a doctor in years. I'm as healthy as a horse." *Uh-huh*, I thought.

Now I'm certain you are thinking, I don't own a prized racehorse, so what's this got to do with me? Sadly, probably more than you realize.

Do you own a pet, such as a dog or cat? If you do, you most likely, like so many others, feed your dogs and pets more carefully than your own kids or yourself.

It's time to re-evaluate your health and fitness philosophy. There's a reason for the statement, "...is as healthy as a horse." Now is the time you should care for yourself like a prized racehorse so you can perform at your best.

- Would you like to have more energy?
- Feel better?
- Have more vitality?
- Look better?
- Improve your overall health?
- Be able to be more active with your kids and grandkids?

If not, you need not go any further because this is not the right weight-loss program for you.

14

THE POWER OF POSITIVE SELF TALK

For things to improve, you have to improve. For things to get better, you have to get better. For things to change, you have to change. And when you improve, everything in your life improves with you."

– Jim Rohn,
World Renowned Motivational Speaker

The Elephant and the Rope

While walking through a circus, a man noticed that the elephant was only secured with a small rope that was tied around one ankle. He wondered why the elephant didn't break free from the rope, as the elephant was certainly strong enough to do so.

Curious, he asked a trainer why the elephant didn't attempt to break free. The trainer explained that they used the same size rope for the elephant when it was a baby. Because it was too small when it was a baby to break free from the rope, *it grew up being conditioned that the rope* is stronger than it is. As an adult, it thinks the rope can still hold it, so it doesn't try to fight it.

The lesson of this story is that the elephant in this case is experiencing a learned response. This phenomenon occurs when someone has been conditioned to anticipate discomfort in some way without having a way to avoid it or make it stop. *After enough conditioning, the person will stop any attempts to avoid the pain, even if they see an opportunity to escape.*

THE NINTH PRINCIPLE FOR HEALTHY WEIGHT LOSS

The ninth fundamental principle for healthy weight loss is to keep a positive mindset.

To successfully lose weight and maintain a healthy body weight for life, you will need to fix the negative self-talk you have been engaging in. If you go through life thinking that you are unable to do something just because you have failed at doing it in the past, you are living with a fixed mindset. You have to let go of your limiting beliefs in order to make the breakthroughs that are required for your ultimate weight-loss success. Don't let other people tell you that you are unable to do something, and don't hold onto an assumption that you are unable to grow and learn from past failures.

Our minds are the most important part of the body for weight reduction, yet it is the one area most weight-loss programs ignore or neglect. Your greatest enemy for reducing weight and shedding those unwanted pounds lives between your ears. Your success in reducing weight begins when you change your mindset. Sandra Yancey, CEO and Founder of the eWomenNetwork, said, "If you want to change what's visible, you need to change what's invisible – your mindset." Sam Milman said, "Thinking about doing something is the same as doing nothing." The same applies to reducing weight. Just thinking about losing weight and not acting is the same as doing nothing to make it happen. Buddha said, "All that we are is the result of what we have thought. The mind is everything. What we think we become."

Your desire to get rid of weight is based on a combination of your thoughts, your feelings, and how those affect your eating habits and actions. This is your mindset. Your feelings lead to your emotions. Your emotions control your thoughts. Your thoughts control your actions. Your actions lead to your temperament. Your temperament determines your behavior, which predicts your results.

Mastering your behavior is paramount to your weight-reduction success. And it all begins with your mindset. Have you wondered why it's so difficult to improve our eating habits? We all know what to do, we just don't do it. The source of being overweight is poor eating habits based on poor choices. So, why do you make poor choices? Perhaps, it's not so much the poor choices we make. Instead, it is our flawed relationship with food. It's from the way we think about food.

Many people turn to food for comfort if they're having a bad day, are hurt, or upset. Do you? In movies or TV shows, when someone is upset or hurt, the first thing they show is that person eating a pint of ice cream or stuffing cookies or cake into their mouth.

Many people enjoy food at social gatherings, holidays, and special occasions such as birthdays and anniversaries. Rarely, if ever, do people think about food as fuel and nutrition for your bodies. Perhaps we just don't care.

The obvious answer to improving our eating habits is to change our thinking about why we eat, what we're eating, when we eat, and how we're eating. Getting rid of the stinking thinking is easy to say, however, not so easy to do. Unfortunately, too many of us have negative thoughts that are non-supportive, and not just for weight loss – it applies to most everything else in life.

Humans have between 12,000 to 60,000 thoughts per day. According to some research, as many as 98 percent of them are exactly ones you had the day before. Talk about creatures of habit! Even more significant, 80 percent of our thoughts are negative. Imagine that – 80 percent of our thoughts are negative and non-supportive.

Take a moment to contemplate what your life would be like if your thought process was reversed, and 80 percent of your thoughts were positive and supportive.

Psychoneuroimmunology is the medical term for the mind/body connection. You've experienced it. We all have. If you've been doing mental work all day, you're likely to feel tired physically, too. Do you come home from work feeling exhausted even though you did not do any physical activity? Contrarily, if you're tired from physical activity, such as manual labor, do you find it difficult to think clearly and focus? That's because there is a direct correlation between how your body feels as it relates to your mind and vice versa.

Negative thoughts are especially draining. Thoughts containing words like "never," "should," and "can't," complaints, whining, or thoughts that diminish your own or another's sense of self-worth deplete the body by producing corresponding chemicals that weaken the physiology.

The good news is, if you can recognize a negative or limiting thought, you can consciously choose to change it. Instead of saying, "I can't lose weight," say, "I have the power to control my weight. I have a strong urge to eat healthy foods and forgo processed foods." The chemicals produced by your body as a response to this kind of thought are more likely to support you in fulfilling your goal.

The only way to override the negative and non-supportive thinking is with positive and supportive thoughts. Rachel Hossie wrote an informative and interesting article for *Insider* titled, "How Self-Talk and One Simple Mantra Helped Me Achieve My Weight Loss Goals for Good" (February 7, 2021). In her article, Rachel talks about her years of failure attempting to lose weight. She relates how she finally was able to lose 35 pounds in six months without going on a diet by changing her mindset. Instead of beating herself up when she would stuff her face with chocolate, drink four glasses of wine, or overeat, she realized you do not have to be "perfect" all of the time. That it was OK to overeat from time to time and that it would not prevent her from achieving her weight-loss goal. All Rachel needed to do was learn from the experience and get back on track.

What Rachel learned was that consistency always trumps perfection and that you are unable to fail if you don't quit. The mantra Rachel used to change her mindset is, "You can't mess this up." She learned this mantra from her personal trainer and life coach, Jordan Syatt. In her article, Rachel writes, "According to psychologist and author of *Chatter: The Voice in Our Head, Why It Matters, and How to Harness It,* Dr. Etahn Kross, my mantra is particularly effective because it uses 'you' rather than 'I.'"

Apparently, Dr. Kross believes that it's a lot easier for others to give advice than to follow their own advice. For some reason by using second and third person pronouns (like "you" or "she"), you are able to be more objective and create some mental distance from your own experiences. Dr. Kross refers to this as "distance self-talk." What this means for you is you are better able to follow through with your goals if you talk to yourself in the second or third person.

In a recent study, Dr. Kross and his team proved this concept with regards to healthy eating.

Rachel pointed out that what you don't see in her before and after photos is the mental work that she has done in her transformation. In her article, Rachel stated, "And that's part of the problem with fad diets or 'quick fixes' – they don't help people develop healthier mindsets, so any physical change that may materialize won't last." And this is another reason that supports the premise that diets don't work.

People who lose weight and get into their ideal shape are focused on the solution. They believe in attaining their goal. They want it and their actions are reflective of their belief. They look for ways to improve rather than reasons why they can't.

The problem for many, especially those who have never really tasted success or know anything else but being overweight is that their belief in themselves reaching their goal is low to non-existent. Their self-esteem sucks. They have terrible, negative, non-supportive self-talk. Do you?

Stop looking outside of you. Everything you need to be successful exists within the space between your ears. You most likely don't need a different gym membership, you don't need a new supplement, and you don't need to follow a new diet. You need to back yourself and BELIEVE! Use affirmations and visualizations as a tool to program your mind to believe and then take consistent and persistent action based on those thoughts.

Stop lying in B.E.D!

B.E.D is Blame – Excuses – Denial. Take responsibility for your thoughts, acknowledge when your self-talk is negative, and then aim to steer your thoughts in a more positive direction. Focus on what you can control and then go take some action based on those thoughts. Realize that your state of consciousness creates your reality, and your reality is yours to make whatever you so choose.

It's imperative that you create the thoughts you want about food and put them on autopilot, so they become second nature and natural. Do it to a point so that your thoughts are no longer negative but are positive. Your positive thinking becomes as normal as brushing your teeth.

If you don't learn to manage your way of thinking about food, you are doomed to a life based in failure and struggle with weight issues. Your old concepts about food will keep you stuck. Consciousness is observing your thoughts and actions so that you can live from true decision-making in the present moment rather than being run by programming from the past.

Let me give you an example. You're at your grandmother's home and just finished a fine meal. Grandma brings out one of her world-famous pecan pies. She knows you want to lose weight. So, she gives you a choice. You can have a piece of the delicious mouth-watering pie or a glass of water.

If you choose the pie, you get immediate joy and satisfaction, an awesome sense of pleasure because the pecan pie is amazing. If you choose the glass of water, you get nothing. And, if the others who joined you for dinner at Grandma's choose the pie, you might feel some anger or resentment. This is the challenge you face. Not just at Grandma's, but every day, all day.

If you make a poor choice by selecting the pie, you're immediately rewarded. You have instantaneous gratification. If you make a good choice, a healthy choice, you get nothing. And that's what you'll be fighting day in and day out. You're fighting against your own mind.

You'll be bombarded with a gauntlet of images and smells designed to increase your cravings and temptations all day long. Your ability to stay focused and disciplined will be challenged by television ads for restaurants, foods, pizza, fried chicken, tempting desserts, snacks, candy, and other things. You'll pass by numerous signs and billboards promoting fast food establishments. Not to mention the occasional office party or get-together with friends.

Here's the paradox. What gives you the short-term instant gratification and pleasure, such as the pecan pie or other foods and beverages, most likely causes you pain and suffering in the long run. You'll be at a higher risk of developing chronic illnesses and diseases such as Type 2 diabetes, different forms of cancer, possible liver disease, and an increased risk for a heart attack or stroke. The other side is that what causes resentment and possible pain, such as choosing to not eat the pie or other desserts, in the short term will reward you in the long term with a higher probability for maintaining a healthy weight and better health.

According to Darren Hardy, in life, you'll "suffer" two types of pain. You get to choose your pain. You can choose the pain of regret or the pain of being disciplined. Hardy said, "The pain of discipline weighs ounces. The pain of regret weighs tons." It's not easy to make the healthier choice. However, it's a lot less painful if the choice of regret is that you do suffer a heart attack, stroke, or contract a chronic illness or disease. The fundamentals of achieving and maintaining a healthy weight are easy: eat holistic (whole) foods, mostly plants, not too much, avoid processed foods, drink lots of pure water, and get proper rest. These, unfortunately, are most often ignored.

It's an internal fight about being consistent. T. Harv Eker said, "How you do anything is how you do everything." Similarly, Dave Ramsey said, "If you live like no one else, later you can live like no one else." Of course, Dave Ramsey was talking about financial advice. However, the same can be applied to achieving and maintaining a healthy weight. If you eat like no one else, i.e., avoid fast foods and processed foods, and eat primarily whole/holistic foods, you'll most likely enjoy good health where others will suffer with chronic illnesses.

It bears repeating: reducing weight is a state of mind. Either you control your thoughts or they control you. Either way, it's your choice. Training and managing your mindset are the most important skills you can learn in terms of both happiness and success. It's doable and you can do it.

A wise man met a group of people who were complaining about the same issues over and over again. Instead of listening to the complaints, he told them a joke, and everyone laughed.

The man repeated the joke. This time, only a few people smiled.

When the man repeated the joke a third time no one reacted.

The man smiled and said, "You won't laugh at the same joke more than once. So, why do you think you will get a different result from continuing to complain about the same problem?"

You are not going to get anywhere with your weight issues if you keep complaining about it yet do nothing to fix it. Instead of wasting your time complaining and expecting other people to continue to react to your complaints, do something to make a change.

Weight-loss programs tend to be a temporary solution because they're incomplete. They don't help people change their thought process or their relationship with food. There is a lot of empirical evidence and data that proves the majority of those who lose weight fail to keep it off. They gain the weight back.

Teaching you how to make improvements and changes to your thinking to improve your eating behavior and habits is extremely important and critical for successfully achieving and maintaining a healthy weight.

What will motivate you to reduce your weight? Or, if this doesn't apply to you, what will motivate someone you know or love who should shed a few pounds, or more, and won't? Anthony Trucks is credited with saying, "The fact that you aren't the weight you want to be, should be enough motivation." Unfortunately, for most of you, it's not.

Each of us has our own word, image, sound, or something that will trigger us to want to slim down. For my friends Henry and Robert, the word "diabetes" scared them so much they finally made a commitment to shed their extra pounds. For other friends, it was being worried about their emerging heart problems. For me, it was my doctor telling me, "Lose weight, or you will die."

The number one reason people decide to lose weight is for health reasons. The second most cited reason for reducing weight is to improve appearances. For others, it might be wanting to look good for a special event, such as a wedding, class reunion, or family photo. Or it may be not wanting to take your shirt off in a pick-up basketball game.

Your mindset matters. Without changing your mindset about weight reduction and a willingness to change your eating habits, any attempt to lose weight and keep it off will be futile. Losing weight is hard. Staying fit and trim is hard, and it never stops. It's like running a marathon without a finish line. Staying fat and overweight is easy.

John F. Kennedy, during his speech at Rice University on September 12, 1962, challenged the American people by saying: *We choose to go to the moon. We choose to go to the moon in this decade and do other things, not because they are easy, but because they are hard; because that goal will serve to organize and measure the best of our energies and skills; because that challenge is one that we're willing to accept….*

You must choose to reduce your weight. You must choose to change your eating habits and lifestyle. Because if you do choose to reduce weight in a healthy and sustainable manner, it will, as Kennedy said, "*Organize and measure the best of [y]our energies and skills.*"

Yesterday You Said Tomorrow

Are you a procrastinator?

Have you put off reducing weight because it wasn't the perfect time, or you struggled with it? Each day, countless numbers of people say they will start their diet tomorrow. Unfortunately, for most of them, tomorrow never comes. Many people will tell themselves, "I'll start Monday." Of course, when Monday rolls around, there's always an excuse for not starting.

Have you used the excuse, "I'll start after the holidays?" Or, maybe, "I'll start after our vacation." Perhaps, you told yourself, "I'll start after we meet our friends for dinner on Wednesday?"

The reality is there is no perfect time to start to improve and change your eating habits and lifestyle. The best advice I can offer you is just start and never stop. As Zig Ziglar so eloquently put it, "You don't have to be great to start, but you have to start to be great."

Nike had a message that really resonated with me: "Yesterday you said tomorrow." We all know that if we put off until tomorrow what we can do today, we are just kidding ourselves. Waiting to do something until tomorrow is another fallacy. More excuses, more justification to delay, until it may be too late. Please don't delay implementing a process to improve and modify your eating behaviors. Act now! You'll either keep making excuses, have reasons, or you'll have results. Another Nike slogan is, "Just Do it." Perhaps it should be, "Just do it now!"

If you wait until you feel like losing weight, you'll likely never accomplish it. Mark Twain stated it best when he said, "Don't wait. The time will never be just right." If you do start a regimen to improve your eating behavior and habits, be certain you are resolved and committed to following through. Half-hearted efforts never produce positive results.

Art Williams wasn't talking about reducing weight when he said, "I'm not telling you it's going to be easy. I'm telling you it's going to be worth it." The same can be said about improving your eating behaviors and habits to lose weight. I can tell you it won't be easy. However, it will be worth it.

Think positively. Watch your thoughts. Watch your words. They have impact. You are not making a sacrifice by avoiding certain foods. You're making a choice. You are not depriving yourself of anything, i.e., sweets, ice cream, cookies, cakes, etc. You're making a choice. Remember, we all make choices. Think positively. Think in terms of releasing weight, rather than losing weight. Think in terms of reducing weight, not losing weight. As I said earlier, when you lose something, you tend to want to find it. You are not foregoing that piece of pumpkin pie or pecan pie. You are making a choice not to indulge.

I'm not telling you that you can never enjoy a piece of cake or pie, or a scoop of ice cream. That is not realistic. If you do decide to indulge and enjoy some ice cream, cake, or pie, only have a small amount. Have a spoonful of ice cream instead of a scoop, or two. Have a sliver of cake or pie. You don't have to eat an entire piece. This can satisfy your craving and not set you back on your weight-loss journey. No one is perfect. If you do overindulge, don't beat yourself up over it. Just keep moving forward.

By the same token, don't keep making excuses for making exceptions. Exceptions tend to become the rule. I'm talking about those little voices in your head telling you, "It's OK to eat that candy bar or cookie," or "You've earned that piece of pie or dessert." No! It's not OK to have that candy bar or eat that cookie. No! It's not OK to "treat" yourself if you're still attempting to lose weight.

Do you want to reduce weight and improve your eating habits or not? If so, what are you willing to improve and change to make it happen? We can all agree nothing about your weight will change if you're not willing to do something different.

It may sound like you're getting conflicting information. You are right. The point you need to understand is, it's not OK to overindulge eating things you know aren't going to help you lose weight. Those chips you're thinking of having, don't. But every so often, if you do have some chips, it's not the end of the world. Just don't make it a new old habit.

Have you attempted to lose weight before only to have someone tell you, "Have just one, it won't kill you?" Or "One cookie won't hurt you." No, it won't hurt you. No, it won't kill you. However, it will prevent you from accomplishing your goal of getting rid of your extra weight. Be polite, but respectfully decline. The word "no" is a complete sentence. Just say, "No, thank you." You do not need to give an explanation. Sometimes I'll tell someone, "It will look better on you than me."

There are many more variations of situations to make an exception so be wary. There will be those people who will tell you, "You can't lose weight, so just go ahead and eat." Or "You won't be able to do it. So, why bother?" Maybe it's your own little voices telling you these negative thoughts. Or you've heard the statistic that 90 percent of those who start a diet fail. And of those who do succeed in dropping the pounds, 85 percent gain it all back. So, why bother?

Have you had those thoughts?

Don't believe them because *they* are the ones who can't. You can do it. Joel Weldon has an expression, "Success comes in cans, not in cannots." You are not dieting. You are improving and changing your eating habits. You are among the 10 to 15 percent who can and will succeed in achieving a healthy weight and maintaining it. You are the exception because you are not participating in the new normal.

The most difficult person to negotiate with is ourselves. We have discussions with the little voices in our head, especially when it comes to reducing weight.

Jerzy Gregorek said, "Hard choices, easy life. Easy choices, hard life." Take a minute to soak that in because this is so true. Hard choices include forcing yourself to act. "Hard choices, easy life" applies to eating healthy now to be healthy later. You're not making a sacrifice by not eating the bread, by not eating the piece of cake or scoop of ice cream. You're not depriving yourself or foregoing anything. It's a choice. You're choosing to not eat whatever it is that's not healthy or helping you to reduce your weight. Hard choices are learning how to do something rather than just waiting for someone else to do it for you. It's being responsible for yourself. It's being accountable – to yourself.

Anyone and everyone can succeed in reducing weight. It comes down to your mind and the little voices we all have. We are all mentally weak when it comes to shedding weight. Our mind is what sabotages us the most. The epic battle of getting rid of your unwanted weight will be won defeating your own mind. Your body can do much more than your mind wants to allow.

The toughest person to negotiate with is yourself. And your potential is much greater than your mind wants you to stretch and go for it. If you are not at the weight you want to be, I'm telling you it's your mind's fault. The reason your mind sabotages your efforts to reduce weight and keep it off is one reason – survival. Survival at all costs. When your survival is threatened, your mind can tap into your raw, awesome potential that you had inside you all along. Outside of survival mode, the mind is weak.

To be more mentally tough when it comes to eating and food choices, scare your brain straight with a threat. Fear is your friend when it comes to stimulating your mind.

Make sure your worst enemy isn't the one residing between your own two ears. It's how you manage that conversation that will determine your success or failure.

The CEO and the Employees – A Story

A CEO of a company, frustrated with the quality of work being done by his employees, started to discipline them for their mistakes or perceived lack of progress. However, nothing seemed to get the employees to improve their work ethics. The employees blamed the CEO for not being promoted to higher-paying positions within the company.

One day, as the employees came into work, they saw a sign on the door that read, "Yesterday, the person who has been holding you back from succeeding in this company passed away. Please gather for a funeral service in the assembly room."

The employees had assumed that the CEO had passed away. And, while they were saddened for the family of their CEO, they were also interested at the prospect of being able to now move up within the company and become more successful.

Upon entering the assembly room, many employees were stunned to see the CEO present. They wondered among themselves, "If it wasn't him who was holding us back from being successful, who was it? Who died?" The CEO asked each employee to pass by the open the coffin to pay their respects. One by one, the employees approached the coffin, and upon looking inside, each was quite surprised. They didn't understand what they saw.

In the coffin, there was only a mirror and a sign. So, when each employee looked in to find out who had been "holding them back from being successful" everyone saw themselves. Next to the mirror, there was a sign that read:

The only person who is able to limit your growth is *you.* You are the only person who can influence your success. Your life changes when you break through your limiting beliefs and realize that you're in control of your life. The most influential relationship you can have is the relationship you have with yourself. Now you know who has been holding you back from living up to your true potential. Are you going to keep allowing that person to hold you back?

You are unable to blame anyone else except yourself if you are not at the weight you want to be. You have to take personal responsibility for your own health – the good and the bad. You are the only one who can be proactive in making improvements to your eating habits.

Do you use declarations each day? Do you use affirmations each day? Declarations are different from affirmations. A declaration is stating the objective of doing something. Whereas an affirmation states that a goal is already happening. This might not be true for your weight-reduction, in which case, your mind will immediately dismiss this statement.

An affirmation is basically just self-talk. It's a statement about ourselves or our situation thaѢs phrased in the present tense as if the self-focused declaration is already true. We continually use affirmations subconsciously with words and thoughts and this flow of affirmations is what creates our life experience in every moment. Blair Singer in his book *Little Voice Mastery* states, "The reason many people never get to their dreams is because they are losing the ultimate 'little voice battle' being waged in their brains."

Did you just think, "What little voice? I don't have a little voice!" That's the one. We all have one. If you're like me and others I know, you probably have more than one.

Behavioral psychologists have proven that more than 77 percent of our self-talk is negative. Have you said to yourself, "Positive declarations or affirmations won't work for me for losing weight?" That's a declaration itself. Just thinking those words is a declaration. And, it has negative consequences. Your perception of being overweight can cause you to gain weight or prevent you from dropping it. Researchers found that thinking of yourself as being overweight can turn into a self-fulfilling prophecy.

According to a 2015 study in the *International Journal of Obesity*, individuals who considered themselves overweight were more likely to gain weight. The study also determined that telling an overweight person to lose weight isn't helpful because it could have a contrary effect. They found it caused more stress for the person, which contributed to that person maintaining their poor eating habits and patterns rather than changing. Remember, one of the primary reasons people overeat and gain weight is because of stress.

Snack mixes, fries, cookies, M&Ms, and ice cream are go-to comfort foods because the high carbs activate the brain's dopamine neuronal reward-motivated behavior. These foods act similarly to an addictive drug that makes you feel better. Again, it all comes down to mindset and how your mind affects your individual eating behavior.

Declarations and affirmations are important for weight loss because they work. Shad Helmstetter, Ph.D. is the author of more than 20 books in the field of personal growth, including *What to Say When You Talk to Yourself* and *Self-Talk for Weight Loss*. Dr. Helmstetter tells of a time when he was overweight and struggling with weight loss for many years. In his story he says he tried every diet imaginable and said all the wrong things to himself, thinking his weight problem would never go away. He says he would diet, lose weight, gain it all back, plus more. Then he'd try another diet and repeat the process.

Dr. Helmstetter said that during his struggles with weight he began to study self-talk. He learned that some professional athletes competing in the Olympics would hire full-time self-talk trainers to keep them motivated. He thought if Olympic athletes could have a full-time self-talk trainer to help them compete for gold medals, then what about the "Olympics of weight loss?" With that thought an idea emerged.

He spent the next several months writing his own affirmations and declarations about his weight loss. Then he recorded them on audio. He'd listen to his affirmations and declarations in the background while he shaved each morning. Morning after morning he'd repeat the process of listening to his voice state his affirmations and declarations.

During the next ten and a half weeks he lost 38 pounds just shaving and playing his self-talk. And he wasn't on a diet. But another interesting and remarkable thing occurred. During the same ten and a half weeks of intentionally listening to his own pep talk and losing weight, his wife was also dropping weight. She'd listen to his words while putting on her makeup while he shaved. She lost 25 pounds. That was more than 20 years ago, and he has never been on another diet since.

Unfortunately, most people engage in self-talk in a negative way. The types of affirmations people use are negative in nature. Do you use words and thoughts intended to build yourself up, or do you gravitate towards things keeping you down? Have you thought, *"Once I lose weight, I'll be good enough"? Or "I'm too fat and ugly now, but when I lose weight, I'll have a boyfriend."* This is Negative Motivation. While negative motivation can provide a short spurt of weight-loss drive, it will ultimately not work out long term. Negative motivation may help you lose 20 to 30 pounds, but you'll likely be mentally worse off than before, and you may even regain the weight you've lost.

To successfully lose weight *and maintain a healthy body weight for life*, you'll need to fix the negative self-talk you've been engaging in. The fix for this is simple. Here is how you can do it:

- Identify the negative self-talk you've been using in your life. (It might help to write these down so that you don't forget them.)
- Create positive affirmations around your negative self-talk. The goal here will be to literally "flip" your negative self-talk into positive affirmations.

Here are some examples:

- *"I am not overweight"* becomes *«I am at my ideal weight.»*
- *"I am losing weight"* becomes *«I am closer and closer to my ideal weight with each and every day.»*

- *"I am not eating junk food or fast food"* becomes *"Everything I eat heals and nourishes my body which helps me reach my ideal weight."*

Get control over your thoughts, over your words and over yourself. It's going to require consistent work to reverse the psychological damage that negative self-talk causes within us. It won't happen overnight. But give it enough time and the weight will melt off.

It's important to use the present tense when you create your new positive affirmations because the present tense will make them feel more sincere, authentic, and genuine. This will accelerate your progress. If you use the future tense such as one day or someday, it puts it off. Make it happen now. "I am…"

If you find yourself thinking or engaging in any negative self-talk, stop yourself. Transform it into the positive, right then and there. Focus on what you do want, not on what you don't want, because what you focus on expands. Here are suggested Weight-Reduction Daily Declarations. These are my personal declarations. You can choose which ones you want to adopt as yours or you can create your own.

1. I am in the process of being slim and fit.
2. I am strong and beautiful at my healthy weight.
3. I am retaining my ideal weight.
4. I eat proper portions. I enjoy using a salad plate instead of a dinner plate.
5. I am an inspiration to others to reduce weight. If I can do it, others can too.
6. I am living a healthy lifestyle and improve each day.
7. My body is a fat-burning machine.
8. I use creative alternatives to keep focused and committed to keeping my weight-reduction goals.
9. I am accountable for my choices.

10. I am resolved to sustaining my reduced weight in a healthy manner.
11. I use positive words with myself and others.
12. My healthy eating habits make me smile with pride.
13. I allow myself to make food choices and decisions for my higher good regardless of what others might say or think.
14. I look and feel terrific. I love my body.
15. I am worry free, stress free, and drama free.
16. I adopt the philosophy, "Your issues are not my issues."
17. My clothes tell me everything about being thinner.

Use "I am" Statements

Affirmations are different from declarations. An affirmation states that a goal is already happening, whereas a declaration is stating the objective of doing something. Staci Danford, a Gratitude Neuroscientist, says you can achieve and maintain a healthy weight using *gratitude*. It must be sincere, and you must believe the words you say.

Below are suggested Healthy Weight Affirmations with *gratitude*. These are my personal "I am" statements. You can choose which ones you want to adopt as yours or you can create your own. Or you can continue to use your declarations because they are similar.

1. I am grateful, appreciative, and happy to be reducing weight.
2. I am grateful and happy to be healthy and fit.
3. I am grateful to be strong and beautiful at my healthy weight.
4. I am grateful and happy retaining my healthy weight.
5. I am grateful to be lighthearted.
6. I am attracting joyful and sincere, loving relationships.
7. I am grateful I eat proper portions. I enjoy using a salad plate instead of a dinner plate.

8. I am grateful to be an inspiration to others. If I can do it, others can too!
9. I am grateful to be living a healthy lifestyle and improve each day.
10. I am grateful my body is a fat-burning machine.
11. I am grateful to be accountable for my choices.
12. I am grateful to use great alternatives to keep focused and committed to my goals.
13. I am grateful to be resolved to sustaining my reduced weight in a healthy manner.
14. I am grateful to use positive words with myself and others.
15. I am grateful my healthy eating habits make me smile with pride.
16. I am grateful to allow myself to make food choices and decisions for my higher good regardless of what others might say or think.
17. I am grateful to look and feel terrific. I love my body.

Let's Recap

The simple elements to achieving and maintaining a healthy weight, according to Dr. David L. Katz, M.D., are:

- Eat holistic (whole) foods,
- Mostly plants,
- Not too much,
- Avoid processed foods, and
- Drink lots of pure water.
- The one additional element I added is to get adequate sleep.

The nine fundamental principles for healthy weight loss are:

1. Drink an adequate amount (64 ounces or more) of pure water
2. Avoid processed and manufactured foods
3. Eat organic, whole/holistic foods, mostly plants

4. Eat slowly
5. Eat small portions
6. Get adequate "quality" sleep (a minimum of 7 to 8 hours)
7. Focus on the food you eat by eliminating distractions that can cause "mindless" eating
8. Give your body 12 to 14 hours, or more, each day to digest and process the food you consume
9. Keep a positive mindset by focusing on the foods you should eat and that are healthy rather than the edible products you crave that are known to be unhealthy. What you focus on expands.

To be successful with anything, you must be able to negotiate and communicate what it is you want. But sometimes the toughest sale of all is selling yourself. It's like when you say to yourself, "I need to exercise today," another voice in your head says, "No, I'm too tired." So, then you say to yourself, "I'll do it tomorrow." Or "I'll do it after work."

Every person who has attempted to lose weight knows that battle. It's the self-talk, or management of it, that will get you through difficult times, or cause you to succumb. Don't let the negativity in, don't let your emotions even get started. Just tell yourself, "No thank you. I've practiced for this situation, and I can control myself." Now you know what to do, and how to improve your eating behavior. The only question is will you? Stop being afraid of what can go wrong and start being positive about what could go right.

15

WHAT YOU FOCUS ON EXPANDS

"What you focus on expands,
and when you focus on the goodness in your life,
you create more of it."

– Oprah Winfrey

Focus on what you want because as Zig Ziglar, world-renowned salesperson and motivational speaker said, "When you focus on problems, you'll have more problems. When you focus on possibilities, you'll have more opportunities." With respect to weight reduction, too many people focus more on being overweight and needing to reduce weight than on the solutions to their overweight issues.

If you're focusing on the fact that you're overweight or fat, then that is what life will keep serving you. In the weight-loss game, those who focus on the problem rather than the solution, get more problems.

People who successfully lose weight and keep it off focus on the solution. They believe in attaining their goal. They want it and their actions are reflective of their belief. They look for ways to improve rather than reasons why they are unable. According to Les Brown, "To achieve something you have never achieved before, you must become someone you have never been."

Everything you need to be successful exists within the space between your ears. You most likely don't need a different gym membership, you don't need a new supplement, and you don't need to follow a new diet. You need to back yourself and BELIEVE!

It's imperative that you create the thoughts you want about food and put them on autopilot, so they become second nature and natural. Do it to a point that your thoughts are no longer negative, rather, they are positive. Your positive thinking becomes as normal as brushing your teeth.

What we focus on we create. Focus on what you want to create rather than what you want to avoid. Think positively. Remember, you are not making a sacrifice by avoiding certain foods. You're making a choice. You are not depriving yourself of anything, i.e., sweets, ice cream, cookies, cakes, etc. You're making a choice.

No one is perfect. If you do overindulge, don't beat yourself up over it. Just keep moving forward.

Bob Proctor, world-renowned motivational speaker said, *"What you think about you bring about."* Applying this to weight loss you could say, "You eat what you think about."

Think about the healthy foods you enjoy eating instead of the unhealthy foods you should not be eating. Here is what I mean. If you think about the candy bar, chips, pretzels, cookies, donuts, or ice cream you shouldn't have, guess what? That will be what you will crave and want to eat. However, if you think about the apple, banana, raw unsalted nuts, or other healthy snacks, then that is what you will crave and eat. If you do this consistently, after a while, you won't think about the junk food. You will have improved and changed your eating habits.

Whenever possible, eat off a blue plate. The color blue is an appetite suppressant, whereas red and yellow are appetite stimulants. That is probably why McDonald's, Wendy's, Burger King, KFC, Carl's Jr., and other fast-food places use red and yellow in their color schemes. The two largest pizza chains, Domino's Pizza and Pizza Hut, both use red in their color schemes.

This is how you can accomplish focusing on what you will eat. Commit to what you are going to eat for the day. You can commit to what you eat for the day either the night before or first thing in the morning. Which ever you pick, always do it the same way. Be consistent. The reason being you are building habits to take the load off of willpower or discipline. You are creating automaticity. What this means for you is you don't need to think about it. It is automatic.

There are three ways to commit:

- Write down or post what you will eat on Facebook or other social media or in a food journal.
- Tell another person via a text message, email, or telephone call, what you will eat. That person can be a support or accountability partner or buddy.
- If you are a religious or spiritual person, make this affirmation: "God/Universe, I commit to eat only and exactly this food (list the food) and nothing else tomorrow/today."

A friend of mine told me a story about his friend Billy. Billy is an alcoholic. He approached his alcoholism by saying, "I'm Billy, and I am an alcoholic. I am sober 28 years. I'm not going to take a drink today. I may very well drink tomorrow. But, today, I am not going to drink." What this means for you is just make one decision, one choice, one day at a time. Commit to what you are going to eat for the day. Write it down. Have a plan and stick to the plan.

Perhaps you can modify Billy's daily recital to be, "I have a food addiction. Today, I will eliminate eating fast food, comfort foods, processed, and manufactured foods. Today, I will eat only real, whole/holistic foods that will nourish my body. I may very well eat fast food, junk food, or unhealthy food tomorrow. However, today I am going to avoid soda, diet soda, fruit juice, and fruit beverages, and drink only water, [or whatever is working for you], because it seems to be working really well. So, I will keep doing it today, beyond that, I have no idea."

The Chef and His Daughter

There once was a girl who constantly complained to her father that her life was so hard and that she didn't know how she would get through all of her struggles. Does this sound familiar to you? She was always tired. She believed that as soon as one problem was solved, another would arise.

Being a chef, the girl's father took her into his kitchen. He boiled three pots of water that were equal in size. He placed potatoes in one pot, eggs in another, and ground coffee beans in the final pot.

He let the pots boil, not saying anything to his daughter.

After twenty minutes he turned the burners off. He removed the potatoes from the pot and put them in a bowl. He did the same with the boiled eggs. Next, he used a ladle to scoop out the boiled coffee and poured it in a mug. He then asked his daughter, "What do you see?"

She responded, "Potatoes, eggs, and coffee."

Her father told her to take a closer look and touch the potatoes. After doing so, she noticed they were soft. Her father then told her to break open an egg. She did so and recognized the hard-boiled egg. Finally, he told her to take a sip of the coffee. It was rich and delicious.

Confused, the girl asked her father, "What does all of this mean?"

The father explained, "Each of these three food items had just undergone the exact same hardship–twenty minutes inside a pot of boiling water. However, each item had a different reaction. The potato went into the water as a strong, hard item, but after being boiled, it turned soft and weak. The egg was fragile when it entered the water, with a thin outer shell protecting a liquid interior. However, after it was left to boil, the inside of the egg became firm and strong. The ground coffee beans were different. Upon being exposed to boiling water, they changed the water to create something new altogether."

He then asked his daughter, "Which are you? When you face adversity, do you respond by becoming soft and weak? Do you build strength? Or do you change the situation?"

Your weight-loss journey will be full of ups and downs, wins and losses, and big shifts in momentum. Adversity will be a big part of your experience. While you would probably rather not encounter any difficulties, it doesn't have to always be a negative thing. You determine how you respond to the issues. Will you let it break you down? Will you stand up and meet the challenge or obstacle head-on? Or will you learn from it to improve your eating habits? What is important to remember is when confronting adversity along your weight-loss journey, you have the freedom to choose how you respond. You can respond in a way that ultimately limits you, or you can choose to have it empower you.

Code of Honor

Do you have a personal Code of Honor?

I'm guessing you probably don't.

A Code of Honor is a set of rules which you and others agree to abide by. It is your principles or a way of life. Without rules, people make up their own.

Thousands of books have been written about diet, weight loss, nutrition, fitness, and exercise. There are numerous weight-loss programs advertised on television, radio, and the internet. At the grocery store checkout, you'll see hundreds of new ideas to lose weight touted on the front covers of magazines. Yet, more than 71 percent of the U.S. adult population is overweight.

How many of you have heard of or have been on the…?

1. Paleo diet?
2. Keto diet?
3. Mediterranean diet?
4. South Beach diet?
5. Jenny Craig?
6. Noom?
7. Nutrisystem?
8. Medifast?
9. HCG, like myself?

10. The Atkins Diet?
11. The Vegan Diet?
12. The Zone Diet?
13. The Ultra Low-Fat Diet?
14. Or the numerous other diets such as the Cabbage Soup diet, the DASH diet, or Raw Food diet

Wow, that's a lot of types of diets. According to Rebecca Stamp in her article published in *The Independent* on January 8, 2020, a poll of 2,000 participants found that the average person will attempt 156 fad diets over the course of their lifetime. The survey was conducted by One Poll and commissioned by Love Fresh Berries. At least 52 percent of the study pool admitted they were confused about which diets were more sustainable than the other. And 20 percent didn't know where to go to get reliable and truthful information about nutrition.

The one thing most diets have in common – they ignore a powerful tool: A Code of Honor.

In his book, ***Team Code of Honor – The Secrets of Champions in Business and Life,*** author Blair Singer states, *"Those who are successful have a very clear Code of Honor that is easy to understand and is not negotiable or subject to interpretations. It's a strong set of rules that everyone around them agrees to and part of what makes everyone around them successful as well."*

To succeed in any weight-reduction program, you'll need a Code of Honor to have rules, to be held accountable, and to have support from others. Make your family, friends, co-workers, colleagues, and even your doctor part of your team to support your weight-reduction journey.

Your Code of Honor reflects you and your standards. Your waistline will determine if you're abiding by your code. Share your code with others. If they are willing to abide by your code, and they agree with it, great. If they disagree with it or aren't on board and willing to help you stick to your code, they may be the wrong fit for you. You might consider re-evaluating your relationship with the people who don't or won't support you.

People without a support team or someone to hold them accountable tend to give up on weight-reduction programs. It is difficult to have a spouse or significant other eating pizza, pasta, or desserts while you're attempting to improve your eating habits. Most people, with few exceptions, need to have someone to check in with to keep them accountable and stay on track.

If you can't find someone to join you on your weight-reduction journey, join or create a weight-reduction meetup group. Having a community that encourages you or one-on-one accountability partner or coach is invaluable.

Your weight reduction Code of Honor is the set of rules *you* agreed to. Every person has their own rules, their own Code of Honor. Therefore, it's imperative that you make sure everyone understands *your* Code of Honor and that you want to play by the rules defined in it and that they must too.

Marines have a strict Code of Honor. They need to be rigid because when bullets start buzzing by a person's head, emotion tends to elevate and intelligence decreases. The code is drilled into Marines over and over to keep them together under pressure. It's a matter of life and death. Otherwise, individuals won't do the right thing to protect the team, the mission, and each other.

I'm not saying being in battle is the same as reducing weight. However, for some of you it can be a matter of life and death. For others, it could make a difference between enjoying life or living in misery.

- Honor your code.
- Respect the code of others.

Here are examples of what you might want to include in your Code of Honor. You can choose which rules you want to adopt as yours or you can create your own.

1. Mission. The mission I have chosen is to reduce weight in a healthy manner and to keep it off!

2. Be accountable.
3. Adjust my relationship with food to ensure it is viewed as fuel for my body and not as comfort from my emotions.
4. Record everything, I ingest in a daily journal.
5. Commit to learning about nutrition and better eating habits.
6. Commit to a lifestyle change.
7. Never impose my standards on anyone else.
8. Never blame others for my failures. I will take 100 percent accountability for my own success. No justifications. I'll either have excuses or results.
9. Be willing to get called out if I violate the code. My team (support group and/or coach) must be willing to enforce the code.
10. Never judge or pre-judge others.
11. Motivate, encourage, and empower others to lose weight, but only if they have a desire to do so.
12. Do not seek sympathy or acknowledgement. I want to reduce weight and keep it off for me. Not anyone else. No one can do it for me. I must be willing to do it myself. Note: It's great if you, the reader, have a purpose or reason, some call it "the why," for wanting to lose weight. But the bottom line is that it's your choice.
13. Don't compare yourself to others. We're all unique; we all have our special gifts.
14. Do not compete with others. Complete others.
15. Be a role model for others.

If you want, add more of what's important to you to your Code of Honor. Take some time to reflect on what's important to you to reduce your weight and keep it off. Share your thoughts and ideas with others before finalizing it. Once you do finalize your Code of Honor, it should not be modified, unless under extreme circumstances.

16

HOW TO FIND AN ACCOUNTABILITY BUDDY OR SUCCESS PARTNER AND WHAT TO DO ONCE YOU FIND THEM

"We become what we think about."

– Earl Nightingale,
World renowned author and radio speaker

An accountability partner or success partner is powerful leverage to help you achieve your weight-loss goals. You have a better chance of achieving your weight-loss goal if you have an accountability partner, success partner, or support buddy. Why? Because many of us value the time, energy, and attention they reserve for us, more than we value our own time. For some reason most of us feel a sense of answerability and obligation to them more so than we do to ourselves.

Without someone to hold you accountable, you are likely to make up excuses and reasons for not following through. However, when another person is involved, you are less likely to make excuses because you don't want to disappoint them or disrespect their commitment to you. For example, if you've hired a personal trainer, you don't want to disappoint them. So, you show up. Otherwise, you would probably find a reason not to workout.

In fact, the American Society of Training and Development did research on accountability. They discovered that people have a 65 percent chance of reaching their goal if they have an accountability partner. The American Society of Training and Development study also found that your chance of successfully reaching a goal increases to 95 percent if you establish an ongoing appointment with your accountability partner.

In a six-month study, published in the *Journal of Consulting and Clinical Psychology*, 66 percent of dieters with a support partner and system were able to lose weight and keep it off, while just 24 percent of those without a support buddy or support system were able to maintain their success. What this means for you is that most diets fail to teach you how to find an accountability buddy or success partner. And, even if they do, they do not teach you what to do.

Finding an accountability partner is easier than you might think. Your accountability partner does ***not*** need to be a mentor or someone who can advise you. Let me repeat that. Your accountability partner does ***not*** need to be a mentor or someone who can advise you. In fact, your accountability partner is not there to advise you at all.

Your accountability partner does not need to be on a weight-loss journey. They don't need to be familiar with your specific eating issues, problems, obstacles, or challenges. Confused?

Here is what you are looking for in an accountability partner:

1. Someone who will commit to showing up on time consistently and without fail.
2. They will show up prepared. They will be brief, and they will be brilliant because you'll teach them what they will need to do to help you.
3. They will hold you accountable. They don't need to know what you should be doing. They only need to know what you said you were going to do last time and hold you to it, saying, "*Last week you said you were going to do X. Did you do it? If not, what are you going to do to fix it?*"

The real magic of having an accountability partner is:

A. Knowing someone else is waiting for you so you've got to show-up. It forces you to stay consistent.
B. Having to tell someone what you are going to do each week forces you to plan better.
C. Having to report your wins, losses, fixes, and aha's at the end of the week has you more aware of your *behavior* progress and weight-loss progress throughout the week.

The accountability meeting, once per week, via phone, Zoom, Skype, or other method needs to only be 15 to 20 minutes.
Here is how to run an accountability call:

Your accountability partner needs to be prepared to ask you the following questions based on the goals and priorities you set for the week:

1. *"What were your top three wins?"*
2. *"What were your top three failures, mistakes, or shortfalls?*

Your accountability partner needs to be prepared to ask you,

1. "Based on your failures, mistakes, or shortfalls, what were your fixes?
2. What will you do to fix your failures, mistakes, or short falls from happening again?"

And, your accountability partner needs to be prepared to ask you, "what were the lessons you learned during the week?"

That's it. Keep it short and to the point. No excuses. Don't waste your accountability partner's time trying to get them to say, "It's OK." You either did what you said you were going to do, or you didn't. If you didn't, focus on what you will do to fix the issue.

17

NUTRITION FACT LABEL/PANEL

"Every time you eat or drink you are either feeding disease or fighting it."

– Heather Morgan,
Actress, Screenwriter, and Comedian

Do you read the nutritional labels on the cans, packages, or boxes of the food you purchase? If you do, do you understand what you're eating?

Do you read the fine print of those delicious low-calorie recipes in magazines? My guess is that you probably don't because most people won't.

In this chapter you'll learn how to read and understand the information provided on the Nutrition Fact label required on all food packaging and the importance of reading the fine print in magazines that provide you with so-called healthy recipes.

Every packaged, or processed, product should have a label. Some restaurants also have nutrition information available. The Nutritional Fact label is also known as the Nutrition Facts panel. It was first introduced in 1993. The Food and Drug Administration updated the food labeling requirements in 2016 to make it easier to see how many calories and added sugars are in a product and to make serving sizes more realistic.

The new requirements took effect January 1, 2021. For now, you may see either the redesigned version or an old version on a product.

The information shown in the Nutrition Facts label is based on a diet of 2,000 calories a day, so you may need to recalculate the percentages based on what you are or should be consuming. You need less than 2,000 calories to reduce weight. Your daily caloric intake should be between 1,250 and 1,500.

How to read and interpret the Nutrition Facts label will be broken down into five steps.

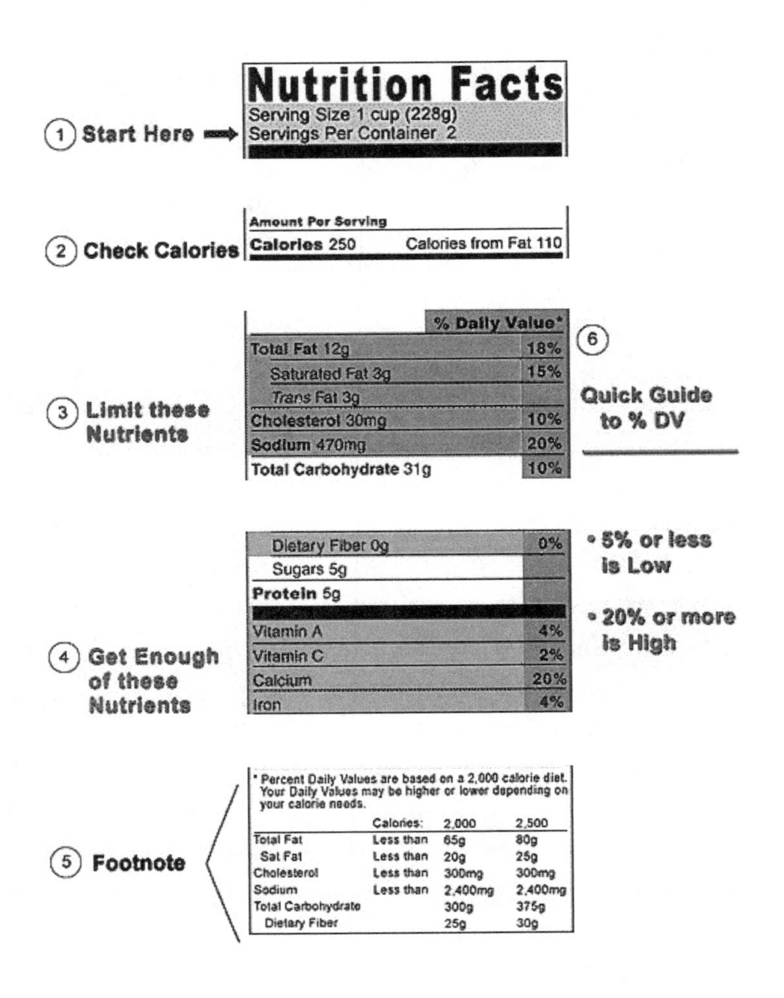

Step One: Start at the top with the serving information. Look at the serving size and the number of servings in the package. Serving sizes are standardized to make it easier to compare similar foods. They are provided in familiar units, such as cups or pieces, followed by the metric amount, such as the number of grams.

The size of the serving on the food package influences the number of calories and all the nutrient amounts listed on the top part of the label. There is a difference between a serving size and a portion. A portion is the amount of food you choose to eat for a meal. Pay attention to the serving size, especially how many servings there are in the food package.

Then ask yourself, "How many servings am I consuming?" For example, a standard 4-ounce can of tuna has two servings. If you eat the entire can of tuna your portion was two serving sizes. That doubles the calories and other nutrient numbers. Instead of 50 calories, you'd consume 100. Your sodium intake would be 180 mg instead of 90.

Step Two: Look at the total calories per serving. Calories provide a measure of how much energy you get from a serving of this food. Many Americans consume more calories than they need without meeting recommended intakes for several essential nutrients. Remember: Your portion amount is based on the number of servings you consume and that will determine the number of calories you eat. As a general guide to calories:

- 40 calories is low
- 100 calories is moderate
- 400 calories or more is high

Eating too many calories per day is linked to being overweight and obese.

Step Three: The Nutrients. Some of the nutrients listed on a label are good while others are bad.

The good nutrients include:

- **Fiber.** Fiber helps your body digest the food you eat. It also can help lower your risk of Type 2 diabetes and heart disease. Food is high in fiber if it contains 5 grams or more per serving. Men 50 years of age or younger should get at least 38 grams of fiber per day. Men over the age of 50 should consume 30 grams of fiber. Women 50 years of age or younger should get at least 25 grams of fiber per day. A woman over the age of 50 should get 21 grams of fiber. Fiber is found in fruits, vegetables, and whole grains. Look for the words "whole grain" on the package and ingredient list versus "multi grain." Multi grain is *not* the same as whole grain.
- **Vitamins and minerals.** The main types include vitamin A, vitamin C, calcium, and iron. Vitamin D and potassium also are important. Talk to your doctor about what vitamins and minerals you need and how much.
- **Fats.** Eating healthy fat is good for your body and will help you to stay satisfied throughout the day. Make sure you're aware of the difference between healthy fats and unhealthy fats. Polyunsaturated and monosaturated promote good health. We'll talk about the bad fats in a moment.
- **Protein.** Protein is important for maintaining muscle mass. When you select foods at the grocery store, read Nutrition Facts labels to choose foods that provide protein. However, the percentage of daily value for protein is not required on the label. Eat moderate portions of lean meat, poultry, fish, eggs, low-fat milk, yogurt, and cheese, plus beans and peas, peanut butter, and seeds.

When you check the nutrition label for protein, scan the fat grams to make sure the number is not too high. Many protein-rich foods are also high in saturated fat, and some foods in the dairy and bakery aisles contain unhealthy trans-fat. Nutrients that are bad for you and which you should avoid or eat less include:

- Fat
- Sodium
- Simple carbohydrates
- Sugars
- **Saturated fat is an unhealthy fat.** This type of fat can increase your risk of heart disease and high cholesterol. The average adult should consume less than 20 grams of saturated fat per day.
- **Trans fat.** This fat also increases your risk of heart disease. Experts could not provide a reference value for *trans* fat nor any other information that the FDA believes adequate to establish a daily value or %DV.

Scientific reports link *trans* fat (and saturated fat) with raising blood LDL («bad») cholesterol levels, both of which increase your risk of coronary heart disease, a leading cause of death in the U.S. Ideally, you should get 0 grams of trans fat per day. Companies can list 0 grams if it contains less than 0.5 grams of trans fat per serving. This means that your food may have trans fat even if the nutrition label says 0.

Check the ingredient list for trans fat products. This includes any partially hydrogenated oil and hydrogenated vegetable oils. Trans fat often is found in baked goods, fried foods, snack foods, and margarine. If you eat more than one serving, you could be eating too much trans-fat.

Cholesterol. You should eat less than 300 milligrams of cholesterol per day. If you have heart disease, aim for less than 200 milligrams per day.

Carbohydrates. Whether or not you're counting carbs, choosing better sources of carbohydrates is important for good health. Instead of simple or refined carbs, eat complex carbs like vegetables, high-fiber fruit, berries, organic short-grain brown rice, and legumes.

Sugars. It's smart to monitor your sugar intake for weight loss and maintenance, as well as overall good health. Selecting foods with a lower number is a good idea. The new Nutrition Facts panel makes it easier to choose healthier options by breaking out the amount of added sugar under the "Total Sugar" heading. Foods with more added sugars provide empty calories and provide very little nutrition. Select foods with fewer added sugars.

Also, check the ingredients to make sure there are no ingredients ending in "OSE" or contain aspartame and other artificial sweeteners. Simple carbohydrates, or sugars, occur naturally in foods such as fruit (fructose) and milk (lactose) or come from refined sources such as table sugar (sucrose) or corn syrup. Added sugars have been required to be on the Nutrition Facts label starting in 2018. The 2015-2020 *Dietary Guidelines for Americans* recommends consuming no more than 10 percent of daily calories from added sugars.

Sodium, or salt, is one nutrient that gets its own bolded line on the label, because too much can be harmful for your health. Most experts recommend that healthy adults limit their sodium intake to no more than 2,300 milligrams per day. If you have a specific health condition, such as high blood pressure or kidney disease, consult your doctor or nutritionist to determine the right amount for you. Low sodium amounts to 140 milligrams or less per serving.

Step Four: Percent of Daily Value. The numbers listed under "% Daily Value" tell you how much a specific nutrient contributes to your total daily diet if you consume 2,000 calories per day. If you consume more or less than 2,000 calories per day, these percentages will not be accurate for you, but they are still useful in making healthy food choices.

Overall, the % Daily Value can quickly help you gauge whether a food is high or low in a nutrient. Generally, a daily value of 5 percent or less means that the food is low in that nutrient and a value of 20 percent or more means that the food is high in the nutrient.

Use the % Daily Value numbers to help evaluate how a food fits into your daily meal plan. Remember, % Daily Value covers the entire day, not just one meal or snack. A food serving with a 5 percent Daily Value of fat provides 5 percent of the total fat that a person consuming 2,000 calories a day should eat.

- You may need more or less than 2,000 calories per day. For some nutrients you may need more or less than 100 percent Daily Value.
- Low is 5 percent or less. Aim low in saturated fat, trans fat, cholesterol, and sodium.
- High is 20 percent or more. Aim high in vitamins, minerals, and fiber.

To summarize:

The % Daily Value tells you the percentage of each nutrient in a single serving in terms of the daily recommended amount for a 2,000 calorie a day diet. If you want to consume less of a nutrient (such as saturated fat or sodium), choose foods with a lower % Daily Value (5 percent or less). If you want to consume more of a nutrient (such as fiber), choose foods with a higher % DV (20 percent or more).

Step Five: Source of Fiber.

Dietary fiber. Fiber is good for you. You'll feel full longer if you eat foods with more dietary fiber. Plus, selecting foods with a higher amount of dietary fiber may help you stick with your new and improved eating behavior. Packaged foods that contain whole grains or vegetables like spinach are often good sources of dietary fiber. Some foods also provide added fiber, which may be helpful for some healthy eaters.

Eating a diet high in dietary fiber promotes healthy bowel function. Additionally, a diet rich in fruits, vegetables, and grain products that contain dietary fiber, particularly soluble fiber, and low in saturated fat and cholesterol may reduce the risk of heart disease.

Consider the additional nutrients listed on the label. You know about calories, but it also is important to know about the other nutrients on the Nutrition Facts label. Make sure you get enough of the nutrients your body needs, such as calcium, choline, dietary fiber, iron, magnesium, potassium, and vitamins A, C, D, and E.*

Note the * used after the heading «%Daily Value» on the Nutrition Facts label. It refers to the Footnote in the lower part of the nutrition label, which tells you **"%DVs are based on a 2,000-calorie diet."** This statement must be on all food labels. But the remaining information in the full footnote may not be on the package if the size of the label is too small.

When the full footnote does appear, it will always be the same. It doesn't change from product to product because it shows recommended dietary advice for all Americans – it is not about a specific food product.

Read the Ingredients!

Vani Hari (*The Food Babe*), *New York Times* best-selling author of *The Food Babe Way: Break Free from the Hidden Contaminants in Your Food and Lose Weight, Look Years Younger, and Get Healthy in Just 21 Days!* and *Feeding You Lies: How to Unravel the Food Industry's Playbook and Reclaim Your Health,* suggests you ask yourself these three questions before eating:

1. What are the ingredients?
2. Are the ingredients nutritious?
3. Where do the ingredients come from?

If you are concerned about your intake of sugars, make sure that added sugars are not listed as one of the first few ingredients. Other names for added sugars include: corn syrup, high-fructose corn syrup, fruit juice concentrate, maltose, dextrose, sucrose, honey, and maple syrup.

Foods with more than one ingredient must have an ingredient list on the label. Ingredients are listed in descending order by weight. Those in the largest amounts are listed first. This information is particularly helpful to individuals with food sensitivities, those who wish to avoid pork or shellfish, limit added sugars, or people who prefer vegetarian eating.

Learn how to read nutrition labels before deciding whether to eat the food or not.

My best advice to you is to eat real food. An avocado or apple will provide you with more nutritional benefits than processed products.

18

FOOD JOURNAL – IT IS MORE THAN JUST COUNTING CALORIES

"What gets measured gets managed."

– Unknown

The most common reason people seem to keep food journals is for weight loss. However, if you want to avoid keeping a food journal, you can commit to what you will eat for the day. You can commit to what you eat for the day the night before or first thing the morning. As you will recall, this was discussed in a previous chapter.

The four most common obstacles to keeping a food diary are:

1. People are embarrassed or ashamed about what they eat.
2. People have a sense of hopelessness, a feeling that it won't help to fill out a food diary.
3. People feel it's too inconvenient to write down what they eat and drink.
4. People feel bad or get upset with themselves when they "slip up."

What can you do to overcome these obstacles and challenges?

Remember that a food journal is an effective tool to reduce weight. There is plenty of empirical evidence, based on research by several organizations, that keeping track of your daily food intake is one of the most effective ways you can change your eating behavior to reduce weight.

In 2009, a group of researchers funded by the National Institute of Health published a study for a different approach to losing weight. They asked 1,600 participants to write down everything they ate for at least one day per week. Notice I said one day per week, not every day.

After six months, those who kept a food log lost twice as much as those who didn't. The researchers learned that many participants started looking at their entries and finding patterns they didn't know existed.

Do you think you can keep track of everything you eat and drink for at least one day per week?

The participants started to implement different behavior modifications that were not suggested by the researchers. Some participants noticed they snacked at 10:00 a.m. so they started keeping an apple or banana in their desk for a midmorning snack instead of hitting the vending machine. Others started using their journals to plan future meals, such as dinner, so they could eat healthier rather than stop at the drive-thru for fast food or junk food in the fridge.

It's been proven that keeping track of what you eat is the most effective method for controlling and reducing your daily caloric, carbs, fat, sugar, and protein intake. Whether you call it a daily food diary, diet journal, calorie tracker, food journal, or diet log, keeping track of your food intake is all about accountability. It's not what you do when someone is watching, it's what you do when no one is watching. Be honest with yourself. Keep your integrity. Tell the truth. Note it in your log if you indulged and ate the slice of birthday cake at the office party. No one is judging you.

According to a study by Kaiser Permanente's Center for Health Research in 2008, keeping a food diary can double a person's weight loss. Their findings were published in the August 2008 issue (Volume 35, Issue 2, Pages 118–126) of *American Journal of Preventive Medicine.* Jack Hollis Ph.D., a researcher at Kaiser Permanente's Center for Health Research, said, "The more food records people kept, the more weight they lost. Those who kept daily food records lost twice as much weight as those who kept no records. It seems that the simple act of writing down what you eat encourages people to consume fewer calories."

The Kaiser Permanente's study was conducted in four cities, Portland, Oregon; Baltimore, Maryland; Durham, North Carolina; and Baton Rouge, Louisiana. In involved 1,685 middle-aged men and women over six months. The average age of the participants in the study was 55.

Food journaling isn't easy or convenient, however, done consistently, it can help you move to more healthful choices. It allows you to keep track of calories, and other aspects of your dietary behaviors and habits. Keeping a food diary/log/record is an important tool in dietary self-awareness, and one of the best ways to improve your eating habits. You can use anything to record your food intake, such as printed booklets, low-tech notebooks or spreadsheets, ready-made apps on iPhones, smartphones, or tablets. Use whatever works best for you.

Kerri Anne Hawkins, a dietitian with Tufts Medical Center's Obesity Consultation Center, uses several types of food diary forms for her patients. She tells them to fill out just what works for them; they can even create their own system – like using sticky notes.

Let's discuss some other basic information to track because it's not just about calories. The food logs we use include an area to track how many glasses of water you drink in a day. This is a great idea because over 75 percent of Americans suffer from chronic dehydration.

Apple Cider Vinegar and Lemon Juice

It is also important to have an area to keep track of drinking apple cider vinegar and lemon juice.

Why?

Because apple cider vinegar and lemon juice have many health benefits. Some of these benefits include:

- Apple cider vinegar helps the body reduce fat
- Apple cider vinegar improves digestion
- Apple cider vinegar balances pH levels
- Apple cider vinegar maintains blood sugar levels
- Apple cider vinegar promotes detoxification of liver

Studies have shown apple cider vinegar:

- Increases metabolism
- Suppresses the appetite
- Helps in oxidation of stored fat
- Contains pectin, a naturally occurring soluble fiber
- It's rich in calcium and potassium – which promote weight loss

By itself, apple cider vinegar does not cause weight loss. However, in conjunction with reducing calories, increased water intake, and improved eating habits, it can help you lose weight. What is important to remember is it will only provide results if used consistently over a prolong time. Be patient.

NOTE: Never drink undiluted apple cider vinegar. Apple cider vinegar should be consumed in water or another liquid because the acid can ruin teeth enamel.

Apple cider vinegar can be used as a salad dressing by mixing 1/2 to 1 teaspoon with 1 tablespoon of extra virgin olive oil and 1 to 2 tablespoons of lemon juice. (Maybe add some ground black pepper and garlic powder.)

The benefits of lemon juice include:

- Promotes hydration
- Good source of vitamin C

- Supports weight loss
- Aids digestion
- Prevents kidney stones

Mix one tablespoon of apple cider vinegar and one tablespoon of lemon juice in eight ounces of pure water in the morning. There is an area on the food log to indicate that this was done.

It's also important to keep track of your sugar intake, how many carbohydrates you eat, and whether they are simple carbs or complex carbs. Contrary to some fad diets, not all carbs are bad. Good carbs are required and necessary for proper nutrition and food balance.

You'll also need to note if you're getting enough protein and fiber. It's important to make sure you're getting enough protein and fiber each day. Most people do not get enough, yet think they do.

What about fats? Are you eating enough healthy good fats and avoiding the bad and scientifically engineered fats?

We shall see.

Be thorough. Note whether a food was fried or broiled; include all toppings, sauces, and condiments. Note all beverages, include cream, sugar, and flavored syrup. And always remember to keep track of portions.

Calories:

To lose a pound each week, you must reduce your intake by about 500 calories per day. For example, if you normally eat 2,000 calories per day, to lose weight you must eat closer to 1,500 calories per day. It is recommended you reduce your calories so that you're eating between 1,250 and 1,500 per day. Reduce your caloric intake gradually.

Keep in mind the average American consumes more than 3,600 calories per day. Here's an example. If you're used to consuming 3,600 or more calories per day, give yourself time to adjust. Again, the goal is to reduce your caloric intake by 500 calories per day until you are comfortable eating less. Counting calories may have a negative impact on you losing weight. The reason being that people tend to overestimate how many calories they burn and underestimate how many calories they consume. Further, low calorie recipes in several magazines may look delicious; however, reading the fine print can be alarming.

There are benefits to monitoring your food intake in other ways than just counting calories.

Many of these low-calorie dishes were loaded with sodium, ranging between 450 to 1,000 mg or more per serving, and/or high carbohydrates, ranging between 35 to 69 grams or more per serving.

As you will recall, it's important to get adequate sleep because the average person, when sleep deprived, will consume an extra 500 calories per day. And to lose one pound you must reduce your caloric intake by 500 calories per day for an entire week.

Can you relate to eating more when you're tired?

Grams of Protein:

You should eat between four and seven ounces of lean protein at each meal. There are about 7 grams of protein in 1 ounce of cooked meat. Eating enough protein is important to losing weight because it's well-supported by science that protein can boost a person's metabolic rate and curb an appetite.

Studies done on protein, as it relates to weight loss, indicate that consuming 25 to 30 percent protein as a percentage of your total daily calories can boost your metabolism by up to 80 to 100 calories per day, compared to lower protein diets.

Protein also can reduce your appetite because it keeps you feeling fuller compared to both fat and carbs. A study done about obese men reported in *Obesity (Silver Springs)* April 19, 2011, issue showed that protein at 25 percent of daily calories increased feelings of fullness, reduced the desire for late-night snacking by half, and reduced obsessive thoughts about food by 60 percent.

In another study reported in the *American Journal of Clinical Nutrition*, July 2005, women who increased their protein intake to 30 percent of their daily calories ate 441 fewer calories per day. The women lost 11 pounds in 12 weeks simply by adding more protein to their diet. It's been found that protein not only helps you lose weight, but it can also prevent you from gaining weight in the first place. In one study reported in the *International Journal of Obesity and Related Metabolic Disorders*, January 2004 issue, a modest increase in protein from 15 percent to 18 percent of calories reduced the amount of fat people regained after weight loss by 50 percent.

According to these and other studies, a protein intake of around 30 percent of calories seems to be optimal for weight loss. This amounts to 150 grams per day for someone on a 2,000- calorie diet. You can calculate how much protein as a percentage of your daily caloric intake by multiplying your calorie intake by 0.075. As an example, if you're consuming 1,500 calories per day, your protein intake should be about 112 grams.

Fried chicken or fried fish does not count as a good source of protein because the oil used to fry the food offsets the benefits. Baked, grilled, or broiled chicken, fish, or meat is the best.

No, a hot dog or bratwurst does not count as a good protein. Again, they are processed foods with too much sodium and nitrates to be beneficial to your weight-reduction endeavors.

Carbohydrates:

Keep your carbohydrate intake between 20 and 50 grams per day. Keep in mind there is a difference between complex carbohydrates as opposed to simple carbohydrates. Avoid simple carbs.

Examples of simple carbohydrates include, but are not limited to, white rice, potatoes, pasta, bread, anything made from grains, bagels, refined sugar, peas, corn, jams and jellies, etc. Note: Although beans and lentils are complex carbohydrates, you should limit the amount you consume because they contain a lot of starch.

Fat:

Between 40 and 53 grams of healthy fat per day is suggested to reduce weight. There are good fats, bad fats, and ugly fats. The good fats are unsaturated fats. Unsaturated fats include polyunsaturated fatty acids and monounsaturated fats. The bad fats are the saturated fats and trans fats (partially hydrogenated fats). Avoid the scientifically engineered fat substitutes such as Olean.

Sugar:

Refined sugar should be avoided. There is no daily requirement for added sugars. Refined sugar doesn't serve any physiological purpose. The less you eat, the healthier you will be. Refined sugar is addicting. Be wary of Starbucks and other specialty shops with trendy or indulgent coffee drinks. Many of their flavored drinks have as much as 71 grams of sugar. According to the American Heart Association, your body needs less than 36 grams of added sugar per day for men and 24 grams for women. A 12 ounce can of Coke has 39 grams of sugar. A 1.55-ounce Hershey's chocolate bar has 24 grams of sugar.

Imagine how many people have a can of Coke and a Hershey bar from the vending machines for a mid-afternoon snack. In other words, you are getting more sugar (refined sugar at that) in one snack than you need for an entire day.

Can you relate to this?

And we wonder why more than 70 percent of the American population is overweight.

Fiber:

Aim for at least 38 grams of fiber per day if you're a male under age 50 and 25 grams if you're a female under age 50 (or 30 and 21 grams daily, respectively, for those over the age of 50). Are you getting enough fiber each day? Are you sure? If you aren't certain you're getting enough dietary fiber each day, track your food intake for a few days or a week.

Fiber is important to reduce constipation. Constipation is a silent epidemic because most people do not want to talk about. Going to the bathroom is a private matter. I'm even uncomfortable talking about this topic.

For many people, constipation is little more than an aggravation. To others it is a daily agony. Few realize that it can be a dangerous and even deadly affliction. But, in 2016, constipation was the reason for six million doctors' visits and 700,000 emergency room visits. This cost billions of dollars in health care costs, along with what Americans spend on over-the-counter laxatives. Chronic constipation can be avoided by changing and improving your eating habits.

Eating a diet with low fiber and lack of enough water causes people to use medications such as laxatives and enemas that can have a negative effect on your bowels.

Can you relate to this issue?

The number of people admitted to the hospital primarily for constipation has more than doubled since 1997.

So, how can you get more fiber in your diet? Here are some suggestions. An avocado has 10 grams of fiber. An apple has 4.4 grams. Those two items alone have 14.4 grams. More than one-third of what you need for a day if you're a man and more than half if you're a woman.

What else should you include in your food log? Rebecca Puhl, Ph.D., director of research at the Rudd Center for Food Policy and Obesity at Yale University, suggests including the location of the meal because these details will provide insight into emotional triggers for eating habits and places where you are most likely to consume healthy and unhealthy foods.

If you're trying to understand how your emotions relate to your food choices, you might also want to include questions in your diary such as, "How hungry am I?" or "What were my emotions before, during, and after the eating episode?"

You should log the details of your food consumption as you go throughout the day or set some time aside at the end of the day to update it. But experts say your record will be more accurate if you do it right after eating. They also say it's important to record everything – even if that seems painful.

While writing in your food journal every day is best, it is not necessary. If possible, write in your food diary at least five days each week. Remember at the beginning of this chapter, you were told that people who recorded everything they ate just one day per week had significant results. Do what will work best for you so long as what you're doing is producing positive results.

And, while it can be tempting to not record a binge episode or eating an impromptu dessert, this is the most important time to track it. Be certain to log in what you ate, why, where, and how much. The reason being it can provide you with valuable insight that can help you change and improve your eating habits.

If you can't bring yourself to fill out a detailed food diary form each day, that's OK. Just writing a minimum amount of information in your food diary will help you in your weight-loss journey. Many people believe that it's necessary to keep a "perfect" food log with every detail, and if they don't, they have failed. It is not necessary or required to keep a perfect food log. Your efforts to record what you eat, and drink get you closer to paying attention to your food choices and habits.

Be motivated and inspired on your weight-reduction journey. In addition to tracking of your food each day, this journal is designed to help you see the connections between your emotions and what you eat, when you eat, and the reason you eat. A simple journal should provide enough information to allow you to see trends that may be causing your weight to stall or gain, an awareness which can ultimately help you accomplish your incremental weight-reduction goals and increase your total weight reduction.

Fill in the journal every day if possible because this will show your connection between food and moods as well as general eating patterns. The more information you fill in, the more patterns you'll see. Change your attitude and your body as you read each declaration or affirmation you learned in the previous lesson.

If you work with a counselor, doctor, or dietician (or are planning to), share your journal with them.

If you find yourself wanting to journal everything you eat in detail, don't. It is not something you should do for the rest of your life. To help you curb the impulse to meticulously chart everything you eat, provide only a small space to record your entries. Allow just enough space to record your meals and snacks in case you run into problems. What is important to remember is you do not need to spend too much time on it. People who recorded their food consumption only one day per week still lost weight.

Drink at least eight 8-ounce glasses of pure water each day. My preference is to drink distilled water. There are arguments on both sides whether this is good or bad. You make your own decision. Pure water is better for you than sodas, flavored water, carbonated water, or fruit juices.

Avoid orange juice and other fruit juices. Fruit juices have too much fructose, glucose, and sucrose. As an example, would you ever sit down and eat four oranges? One orange is plenty. But it takes four medium oranges to make an 8-ounce glass of orange juice. Juicing removes the fiber and gives you 28 grams of carbohydrates.

Questions to keep in mind as you complete the food journal:

1. Are certain foods causing mood swings?
2. Do you use food to improve your mood or energy?
3. Are there certain times of the day or situations when you're susceptible to cravings?
4. Out of habit do you associate certain activities with eating, such as watching TV, eating popcorn at a movie theater, etc.?
5. Does an increased level of stress cause you to eat more?
6. What types of food do you crave?
7. Is too much caffeine causing anxiety or mood swings?

Food for Thought – Things to Ponder and Contemplate to Gain Insight into Your Eating Habits

Dr. Joseph Mercola, in his book, *Fat for Food Ketogenic Cookbook,* stated, "...when Hippocrates wrote, 'Let food be thy medicine and medicine be thy food,' he shared an elemental truth: if your food isn't contributing to your health, it's contributing to your illness."

Note the time and location, and your mood and satiety, to help you identify patterns and triggers. Why are you eating a mid-afternoon bag of chips? How much of your caloric intake occurs while you are watching TV?

Time:

Writing down when you eat helps you to see if emotional eating happens at specific times. Is your eating hunger-driven or is it because you're emotional? If possible, the best time to eat your meals is between 7:00 a.m. and 7:00 p.m. Some advocate for a smaller window to consume your food. However, with a 12-hour period, it gives your body 12 hours to process and digest your food.

Why are you eating?

Are you stressed? Anxious? Upset about something or someone? Do you eat when you're nervous? Are you eating when you're lonely or sad? Do you eat when you're bored? Are you eating for comfort? Or, are you consuming food as fuel for your body? Emotional eating can be modified and altered once you're aware that it's happening.

Here are reasons people gave as to why they ate:

1. I ate when I was bored.
2. I ate when I'd watch television.
3. I ate when I was worried or stressed.
4. I ate when I was frustrated or upset.
5. I ate to reward myself.
6. I ate to make myself feel better.
7. I ate because I was lonely.

You might be able to add a few reasons of your own.
Did you notice what all the reasons have in common?
Give up?

Not one reason given for eating was for nutrition or for fuel for your body.

All animals in their natural state, except for humans, eat ***only*** for the purpose of maintaining health and nutrition. Humans are the only species that eats for pleasure and comfort.

According to Dr. Shad Helmstetter, "We overeat to fulfill the needs of the mind."

The reason you should eat is for nutrition and as fuel for your body. Keep this in mind when you are recording what you are eating. Because it's just as important to understand why you are eating as what you are eating. Once you understand that eating should be to provide fuel and proper nourishment for your body, you'll have a different perspective about food.

Can you see how your perception about food could change and improve your eating habits?

What Types of Foods Are You Eating?

Writing down what you eat helps you see connections between moods and certain foods. Are you tempted to eat cookies or ice cream when you're stressed? Or do you reach for a candy bar when you're nervous? Maybe you prefer salty foods such as potato chips, pretzels, or something crunchy if you're feeling lonely or sad? Are you eating foods that satiate you or just lead to more cravings? Are you getting any protein?

Environment:

Does what's happening around you affect your eating? Some people tend to snack when watching TV. Others turn to food if other family members are eating too. Where are you eating? At the kitchen table? While watching TV? In your car driving? At your desk in your office or at work? A restaurant? Does where you eat increase the quantity you consume? If so, you might consider consciously changing the location of your meals.

Watching television detrimentally affects your eating habits, which can cause obesity. Studies show a direct correlation between watching television and weight gain. People tend to snack on calorie-dense processed foods while viewing the boob tube. Studies have shown that viewers consume 65 percent more calories from snacks while watching television.

In Chapter Eleven, you read about eating while watching television, and not just the taste temptations, but how TV commercial tactics can trigger your desire to eat, whether it is a desire for food or comfort.

This bears repeating: One study found 34 percent of viewers were more likely to order high-fat, high-sugar foods from menus than those who didn't watch television. Who wants to order a pizza from Pizza Hut, Little Caesars, or Dominoes? Perhaps by keeping a food journal you'll discover you're watching a lot more television than you thought.

In Chapter Eleven, you read tips for things to do to combat a television eating habit, such as push-ups, leg-lifts, or working with dumbbells. In other words, giving yourself a mini-workout. It's a great distraction. You could even walk briskly around the house. You don't need to sit like a lump in front of the TV for hours, and this way you can get a little exercise, ignore the messages bombarding your senses, and perk up your brain.

You might consider tracking how many hours you spend watching television. It may surprise you how much time you're wasting in front of the screen.

Track and record your eating behavior for a few weeks. Then look for patterns. If it appears there's a relationship between eating and feelings, think of ways to meet the emotional needs without turning to food. Ask people in the support community for suggestions. Or ask if they will be an accountability buddy you can talk with to avoid comfort eating. Maybe take a walk, do some yoga or quick exercise. Find other ways to deal with frustration.

Starting a food journal is one thing. Sticking with it is another matter and ideally, it's something that should be done for weeks rather than days. The medical literature talks about non-compliance and that many people will only record in a journal for a few days or only a week and give up. "Food journaling is hard," said James Fogarty, associate professor of computer science and engineering at the University of Washington in Seattle. Dr. Fogarty and co-researchers have explored the barriers to keeping a food journal by examining several online food journal websites to see how design might influence the difficulty people often find sticking with them.

Here's a little advice from Jim Rohn on keeping a journal for the past 40-plus years:

> *"Be a collector of good ideas, but don't trust your memory.*
>
> *The best collecting place for all the ideas and information that comes your way is your journal.*
>
> *The reason why I spend so much money for my journals is to press me to find something valuable to put in them.*
>
> *"Don't use your mind for a filing cabinet.*
> *Use your mind to work out problems and find answers,*
> *file away good ideas in your journal."*

19

LEARNING BY TRIAL AND ERROR: WHY LEARNING FROM OUR MISTAKES IS IMPORTANT

"What makes me happy is seeing the evidence of weight-loss progress on others."

– David Medansky,
The Overweight Person's Best Friend

In the opening scene of *Batman Begins* (2005), Thomas Wayne asks his son, who has fallen into a dry well, "Why do we fall, Bruce? So that we can learn to pick ourselves up."

Toward the end of *Batman Begins*, Michael Caine, playing Alfred Pennyworth, says to Christian Bale, playing Bruce Wayne, "Why do we fall, sir? So that we can learn to pick ourselves up."

We all make mistakes. However, the question is, did you learn from your mistakes?

Can we agree that we all learn by trial and error? Learning by trial and error is how you can figure out what will work for you and what won't when it comes to achieving a healthy weight.

Do you realize that it is better to learn from the mistakes of others rather than your own mistakes? We'll get to the reason in a moment. In the meantime, it's important to understand that the one mechanism humans have developed to avoid making the same mistake over and over is the spoken word, the written word – otherwise known as language. The word is a shortcut to passing along information from one generation to the next, because words convey concepts.

R. Buckminster (Bucky) Fuller wrote an article for *Intuition* magazine titled "Mistake Mystique" that connected language and mistakes to learning. Bucky Fuller was a 20th century inventor and visionary who published more than 30 books. Fuller did not limit himself to one field but worked as a "comprehensive anticipatory design scientist" to solve global problems. Fuller's ideas and work continue to influence new generations of designers, architects, scientists, and artists.

One notion gleaned from the "Mistake Mystique" article is that in addition to the basic needs of food, water, shelter, and nurturing, we need to be curious to learn. He said being curious to learn is a basic human need. Fuller surmised that to survive as a species, it's necessary to multiply and to develop words as a short cut to explain concepts to help future generations to avoid the same mistakes.

Let me provide an example to illustrate this point. Imagine you travel back in time to ancient Rome. How would you communicate the concept of an automobile, an airplane, or a rocket ship? Today, you can do this using one word. You can understand what is being communicated to you when you hear the word automobile, airplane, or rocket ship. We may have different visualizations of what is being conveyed, however, the concept is understood. On the other hand, back in ancient Rome, you'd need more words to convey the concepts of these modern-day terms.

Life is a journey full of making mistakes. And that's a good thing, so long as we learn from them. The word "mistake" unfairly means something bad or negative. This is a misconception.

The definition of "mistake" is an action or judgment that is misguided or wrong. Just because it is incorrect, does not make it bad. In the movie

National Treasure, Nicolas Cage, playing Benjamin Gates, said, "*You know, Thomas Edison tried and failed nearly 2,000 times to develop the carbonized cotton filament for the incandescent lightbulb. And when asked about it he said, 'I didn't fail. I found 2,000 ways how not to make a light bulb,' but he only needed to find one way to make it work.*"

Edison didn't look at the mistakes of finding the correct way to make the carbonized cotton filament as bad or negative. He saw them as learning opportunities, and so can you. What is wrong with making a mistake if that is how we learn? Being wrong about something does not necessarily translate into it being bad or negative. It's important to view a mistake, miscalculation, misunderstanding, oversight, or something misconstrued as a positive, a learning opportunity to figure out the one way or several ways to get it right.

This applies to weight loss. There are many ways to lose weight and keep it off. You only need to figure out the one way for you to reduce weight in a healthy manner that you can sustain.

Hollywood gives a great explanation for why "miss-takes" are valuable. In filming a movie or TV series, Hollywood uses a clapperboard to mark the beginning of a segment for editing purposes. A clapperboard makes a loud sound. It's used in filmmaking and video production to help synchronize the picture with the sound or audio. It also designates the various scenes as they are being recorded. Each scene or "shot" is numbered, starting with "take one" and continuing until filming is completed.

A miss-take (missed take) or outtake is a scene not used in the edited version of a film or videotape. In other words, a mistake. Actors and directors do many takes to get the scene right. They're learning from mistakes to get the scene correct. They do many takes before getting it right. So why should a mistake be viewed or construed as "bad" or a negative if it's a learning tool used in Hollywood?

Unlike Hollywood, teachers can stunt a child's learning development by punishing them for a mistake. If you make an error answering a question on a test, you're marked down. This doesn't encourage students to learn from their mistakes as would the ability to re-take the exam or quiz and get credit for realizing what they did wrong. Haven't we agreed that learning comes from making mistakes and correcting ourselves? How does it help a child learn to make them feel "bad" if they do poorly on a test or quiz? It doesn't. The only thing a child learns is that it's "bad" to make a mistake.

We learn by trial and error. Your best teacher is your last mistake. Are you willing to admit your mistakes when it comes to reducing weight, so you can learn and achieve your goal or objective more quickly?

We all make mistakes every day. However, you still might not view them as learning opportunities. In this chapter you'll be taught several powerful lessons you can acquire from making a mistake.

1. **A mistake teaches you to clarify what you really want and how you want to live**. The word "mistake" gets its meaning from you. You give it meaning. The word "mistake" can be perceived differently by each person. How many of you compare "mistake" with success?

Noticing and admitting your mistakes along your weight-reduction journey helps you stay in touch with your commitment – what you want to accomplish and what you need to do to shed those unwanted pounds.

A mistake is like a flashing sign that says, "improve or change this." The urgency is to focus on the obstacles or challenges preventing you from making different choices when deciding what to eat or which beverage to drink. Re-examining why we made a choice to indulge can help get you back on track, provide clarity, and help stay positive to improve next time the situation occurs.

2. **A mistake teaches you to be honest with yourself.** It's natural to want to hide our mistake if we eat what we know we shouldn't – like a slice of pizza or several pieces of bread served at the restaurant because we get embarrassed by a lack of discipline. However, being honest with yourself is an opportunity to improve

the next time. It's like holding up a mirror to yourself and really seeing. What you do in private, you wear in public. You're not fooling anyone other than yourself. Here's an exercise you can do when this happens:

- Ask yourself what happened? (I ate some bread).
- How did it make you feel? (I felt guilty).
- What can we learn from this experience? (Be honest with the decision and not hide it).
- How can you use what you learned in the future? (Avoid bread at the restaurant by asking the server to not bring any or keep it at the other end of the table, or drink water instead of munching on the bread.)

Being honest with yourself will help you concentrate on letting go of the embarrassment to learn. It's not what you do when people are watching, it's what you do in private when no one is watching – except yourself.

3. **A mistake will teach you to accept your fallibility**. Sometimes even your best efforts just don't work out. We all have good intentions to lose weight. You might have tried a diet and failed and tried another and failed again. When this happens, admit you're stuck. Ask for support. Ask someone to keep you accountable. When you admit you're stuck and are unable to do it alone, it sends a signal and opens the door for help to show up. Solutions, resources, even a person might appear in your life to help you resolve your being overweight issue.
4. **A mistake can teach you**, through analysis and feedback, what's working and what's not. It's your reality check. By making a mistake, you'll learn what doesn't work on the path to reducing weight and learn or find out what will work for you. The feedback you get from your mistake can be the most specific and meaningful

information you'll receive. Often, you can trace a mistake to a behavior or belief that can be changed and improved. Maybe you'll have that "aha" moment by filtering your mistake through a series of questions: How can I use this experience to improve? What will I do differently next time? How will I be different in the future? Questions like these lead to an inquiry that invites solutions.

5. **A mistake can teach you to be accountable**. Our instinctive reaction when we make a mistake is to shift blame rather than accept responsibility and learn from it. It's more empowering for you to accept your role in making a mistake, learn from it, and move on. Shifting the blame to others won't help you. Remember, it's about understanding what you can do differently next time. Delving into the mistake instead of ignoring it or shifting blame reminds you that you have choices, and your actions have a huge influence on your weight-loss success. Anything is possible. You have options. I respect your choices. Keep in mind, Emerson said, "Your actions speak so loud I cannot hear what you are saying."
6. **A mistake says a lot about your integrity**. A mistake will often happen because you break your promise, overcommit, or agree with someone else's agenda to avoid conflict. How many of you promised you'd lose weight? How many of you kept your promise? How many of you committed to exercising more or eating more fruits and vegetables? How many of you said you'd eat less processed food? These are examples of breaking a promise or overcommitting.

By now, hopefully, you'll have started to implement the weight-loss principles you were given in the previous chapters.

Big mistakes generally start as small errors.

Gaining weight starts by making choices to eat differently. It's more convenient to pick up food at a drive-thru than prepare a meal at home.

We're tired, hungry, and we become complacent. Over time, these tiny choices accumulate and show on our waistline or cause a medical ailment, debilitating illness, or disease.

When we maintain our integrity to improve our eating habits, we pay attention to the choices we make each day. The nearer we live to the source of health, the more health we shall receive. A mistake can be a signal that that our words are out of alignment with our actions. If this happens, you can re-examine your intentions, reconsider your commitment, and adjust your actions.

Your history does not predict your future. Anything is possible. You have options. I respect your choices. When confronted with making a mistake while attempting to reduce weight, do you pull back, retreat? Or do you rise to the challenge, figure out a way to overcome the obstacle preventing your weight loss, and move forward?

Your mistake can inspire others. Were you inspired by my weight-reduction story of shedding 50 pounds in four months? Are you inspired by others who are successfully dropping weight? Does that inspire you to commit to doing the same?

Let's examine how failure can help you with your weight-loss journey. We've all *experienced failure at some point in our lives.* J.K. Rowling said, "It is impossible to live without failing at something, unless you live so cautiously that you might as well not have lived at all, in which case you have failed by default."

Failure is defined as a lack of success; the fact of not doing something that you must do or are expected to do. According to the English Oxford Dictionary, failure is a lack of success, the neglect or omission of expected or required action, the action or state of not functioning. So why is failure necessary to be successful? Because failure is like a mistake. It is through your failures that you can learn your greatest lessons in life.

Do you think about failure in a negative light?

Yes, failure is painful. Yes, it causes emotional turmoil and upset. Yes, it inflicts agonizing pangs of shame, grief, and distress. However, those who have bounced back from true failure, understand that failure is necessary for success. If you're not tested by adversity, you might not realize your full potential. If you're not tested by adversity to reduce weight and shed your unwanted pounds, you might be content to remain overweight.

Being overweight is failure. It is failure of not drinking enough pure water and eating healthier. Yet, your failure can help you find your determination to successfully lose weight and keep it off.

Here's an example. When a baby is learning to walk, it will fall down often. This is failure. But every mother knows that their baby will walk one day. The baby will fall down many times, but it will walk. Why is a mother so confident that her child will walk? Because, as we all know, falling down and failing while learning to walk is just a part of life. It's normal to learn from our failure. It's like riding a bicycle. Were you able to hop on a bike and ride it the first time? Unless it had training wheels, probably not.

What we don't realize is some people, like me, had to go through the experience of gaining and losing weight, to get to where they are in life as it relates to weight. Let me explain. Like many of you, I wasn't always overweight. I was fit and trim. However, as with many of you, life happened. Before I realized it, I had gained a lot of weight. I had to experience the failure of gaining weight to experience the success of reducing weight.

If I hadn't gained the weight, I could not relate to you when you tell me what it feels like to be overweight. I couldn't relate to you when you tell me how it feels to be embarrassed by your weight. Or, how it feels to fail to lose weight after turning from one diet to another. To succeed, I had to fail. Now, I'm driven by my fear of failure to maintain a healthy weight. After all, how would it look for a weight-reduction specialist to be overweight?

Here's the rub. Society tends to celebrate the success rather than highlighting the heroic journeys achieving success, the setbacks, upsets, and failures it took. It's not glamorous to talk about getting fired from a job only to succeed in starting a business. It's not appealing for me to look at photos of myself when I was overweight. Rachel Gillet wrote, "What may initially feel like failure may just be the launching pad needed for success."

J.K. Rowling, when she was a secretary for the London office of Amnesty International, spent too much time at work writing about a teenage wizard named Harry Potter. Rowling secretly wrote her stories on her work computer and daydreamed about being a writer. Her employer got fed up and terminated her employment. Her severance check helped support her over the next few years. The original *Harry Potter* manuscript was rejected by 12 publishing houses before Bloomsbury picked it up.

Michael Jordan expressed failure another way: "I've missed more than 9,000 shots in my career. I've lost almost 300 games. 26 times, I've been trusted to take the game winning shot and missed. I've failed over and over and over again in my life. And that's why I succeed."

So, are you ready to learn from your weight-loss failures, otherwise known as diets, to modify your lifestyle and improve your eating habits?

Think of failure as a stepping-stone. You'll learn several powerful life lessons that failure helps to instill in us and teach. If you've failed to lose weight and keep it off, and you're going through a rough time right now, keep these important lessons in mind.

An important lesson gained from failure is experience.

What happens when you fail? You gain first-hand experience. Your journey through life is based on your experiences. Failure brings you knowledge that can be used for future situations.

Failure in life builds resilience.

The more you fail, the more resilient you become. For you to achieve weight-loss success, you must know how to be resilient. If you think you're going to succeed at reducing weight the first attempt you make, you're mistaken. Resilience is being persistent. You must be persistent to reduce weight, to keep making improved food choices. To keep moving forward when you have an off moment or day.

Failure creates value.

In thinking about your past failures, think about how much value you bring with you to the table. You're able to share your knowledge gained from your past failures and that make you valuable.

Once you comprehend the value of failure and how it's meant to serve you rather than hinder you, your mind and heart are open to experience failure. Ultimately, you'll have to decide what is failure. What you might consider a failure, say, losing 20 pounds, another might see that as a success. But it doesn't matter how others view your weight-reduction journey. What matters is how you view it and what you consider success.

When you reach a plateau and haven't lost as much weight as you set as a goal, there will be people telling you, "I told you so," and "I knew you wouldn't do it." Maybe one of those voices is in your own head. Ignore these people. Be resilient. Be persistent. Keep making those small adjustments consistently to your daily eating routine. After a few months, you'll see noticeable results. Those who said you couldn't or wouldn't do it will be envious of your results.

It's OK to fail. But it's not OK to give up. Success will taste so much sweeter when you reach your healthy weight. You'll look and feel amazing in that new outfit. You'll have more energy and be more confident. Failure might take you on a path you might not want to travel on. But, the truth of the situation is that path will help shape you into a better person, a healthier person. Unfortunately, there is no path forward in life without experiencing failure. It's what you do with experiencing failure and applying the lessons learned that will determine your ultimate success.

Let's review how to debrief after failure.

- First, determine what happened. The facts.
- Next, how did this make you feel? Your feelings.
- Then, what did you learn from this failure? The findings.
- And, how can you apply what you learned from the failure to future situations or events? The future.

Your being overweight is a failure to eat healthy. And let me reiterate right here: It is not a failure as a human being, it's just a failure to eat healthy. And you can do something about that. Your being overweight and learning to eat healthier can be a great platform for personal development that is unmatched.

Without my being overweight and having to shed my unwanted and unhealthy pounds, I'd never have met the people I've met, been able to help so many other individuals reduce weight and learn to spot the weight-loss rhetoric being spewed by people wanting to take advantage of others for a profit. If you firmly believe in your weight-reduction goals, you can use the lessons learned from failure to push past your old limitations. Thomas Edison said, *"If we did all the things we are capable of, we would astound ourselves."*

20

CONSISTENCY

"It is easier to stay in shape than it is to get in shape."

– Will Smith,

Actor, film producer, and four-time Grammy Award winner

BE RELENTLESS.

Develop a dedicated consistency to your better you. Be unreasonable. Be uncompromising. Go the extra mile. It is the extra mile where success is achieved. Make the extra effort, spend the extra time and preparation to be healthier. Extra is what will separate you from the average person. It is the "extra" that goes in front of "ordinary" to make you extraordinary. And realize, you will make mistakes. No person is perfect. Keep going. Be persistent. That will separate you from those who successfully reduce weight and those who fail.

CONSISTENCY

Consistency is one of the important principles of your weight-loss success. You can improve your health by changing your eating routines and food choices. Your improved eating routines and food choices become your new eating behaviors. Your new behaviors repeated become new habits. Eating habits compounded over time has a direct correlation to your health. Aristotle said, "We are what we repeatedly do." If you ever want to improve your health, you will need to change your daily food choices.

Lack of consistency will derail your weight-loss success. The start and stop process of diets kills the progress of your weight-loss pursuit and permanent results. Healthy and sustainable weight-loss success is about getting you to do what you know needs to be done consistently and permanently. After all, most of us know what to do to eat healthy. We just don't do it.

Consistency is the single most important predictor of weight-loss success. You can accomplish what seems incredible, extraordinary weight loss results in short spurts. However, if your improved eating habits are not continued, eventually it is all for nothing. Perhaps that is why more than 90 percent of people who lose weight on a diet gain it all back, some even more.

What is important to remember is that consistency can work for you or it can turn against you. Consider this: Many people would rather eat pizza every Saturday night for an entire year without thinking about the weight they are gaining. Then, they are shocked when they weight 5, 10, or 15 pounds more than the previous year. However, if you consistently chose not to eat pizza every Saturday night, you might not gain those extra pounds.

Here is an example of why consistency is so important to your weight-loss success. You've decided it is time for you to do something to lose weight. You are going to change your eating habits. You are going to change your lifestyle. You are excited. You declare to yourself and everyone what you are going to do.

You start on your new eating routines. You go for an entire week. You get on the scale expecting to celebrate your new weight-loss success. Except, the scale has not moved. Nothing. You haven't lost a pound. You look in the mirror and you don't see any change whatsoever. Your clothes still fit the same. This is when most people quit.

That is why most people who make a New Year's resolution to lose weight and get in better shape give up by late January. It is called *discouragement.* All your effort and no results. This is when you need to have faith, to trust the process. What is important to keep in mind is that the butterfly soars because it trusts the process of change. You unknowingly have started the compound effect. However, the results are too small and remain invisible for now.

Just keep eating healthy and making good food choices. And, let's say you do this for another three to four weeks. Much to your horror, you have only shed a few pounds. Not like the television commercials that promise, no, guarantee, that you will lose up to 20 pounds in just one month. This is when other people really get frustrated. When, for example, after four weeks you have only shed a few pounds. You have said "No" to all the nachos. You have declined to eat all of the snacks, foregone all the candy bars, and resisted the cookies at the office or other places. This is when another large percentage of people quit. And, you might be here in your own weight-loss process.

However, you keep the faith and trust the process. You remain consistent in your improved eating routines and behaviors. Now you start to see that your clothes are feeling a little looser, or you have more energy, more mental clarity, or just overall feel better. It is easier to keep consistent than it is to start over. If you slack off for even a few days or for a week because you went on vacation, or because of work deadlines, or the holidays, your old habits take over. All of the progress you have made is gone.

Don't believe me? Why do you think more than 90 percent of people who lose weight on a diet gain it back? It is because they revert back to their old eating habits and poor food choices. It will take all that hard effort of seeing no results for a while just to get back to where you were. Will Smith, when asked what he did to get into shape for his roles in movies said, *"It is easier to stay in shape than it is to get in shape."*

It is important to remember that the average person will attempt 126 fad diets during their lifetime. Albert Einstein said, "The definition of insanity is doing the same thing over and over and expecting different results." The definition of weight-loss insanity is attempting diet after diet and expecting different results. After all, diets are designed to fail.

The big secret here is to not stop your improved eating routines. Researchers in London found that it will take, on average, as long as 66 days to develop new habits. What is important to remember is that routines done consistently for a long period of time turn into behaviors. Behaviors done consistently for a long period of time turn into habits. This is one reason why old habits are so difficult to break and new habits are so hard to create. And that is the rub. It is difficult to maintain and keep those good healthy eating habits and so easy to return to the bad unhealthy habits.

You need to master consistency, because if you remain consistent, it is easier to keep the weight off. We are an accumulation of what we do over time. However, we all drift. The difference between those who are able to keep the weight off and those who don't is the ones that keep it off adjust. They recalculate. Just as the pilot in the plane is always adjusting and recalculating its course.

Along with consistency is momentum. Momentum is powerful. Unfortunately, it is tragic if you lose your momentum. Think of a locomotive. It takes a massive amount of energy to get a train off a dead stop to move two inches forward. If you put a two-inch block in front of its wheels, no matter how much steam and energy you give it, the train will not move forward. It will remain blocked.

On the other hand, once you get that iron horse moving and it settles into a consistent rhythm, it gets into that elusive force known as momentum. And once in momentum, in that mode, it becomes nearly unstoppable. Instead of that two-inch block, you can set a concrete steel reinforced barrier on the track and it will rip through it like crêpe paper.

The takeaway here is that once you are in momentum on your weight-loss journey, it requires a lot less energy to keep moving in the right direction. This is where you want to get your daily eating routines, your patterns, behaviors, and habits – into momentum. However, if you let your momentum dwindle, and your locomotive slows or comes to a complete halt (because you might have taken that two-week vacation, got busy at work, chose convenient processed and manufactured foods, ordered take-out or ate fast foods, for a while, especially around the holidays), it will require you to stoke that boiler once again with massive amounts of steam to get back to where you were. You are unable to afford to lose momentum. Once you get momentum, don't lose it.

So, how do you get and keep momentum? According to Darren Hardy, *"Momentum is created through the rhythm of systematized routines executed consistently."* What this means for you is you need to have a system to achieve your weight-loss destination and a system to keep it off. You want systems instead of goals. Losing 15, 20, 30, or more pounds is a goal. Learning to eat right is a system. Having a goal is not going to help you to lose weight. The system to achieve the goal is what you want to focus your energy on. People tend to focus on their problem of being overweight instead of the solution to shed the weight.

Systems will always outdo goals. Whatever your weight-loss or fitness goals may be, make sure you have a system to achieve the goal. Then focus on the systems not the goals. In other words, focus on the process rather than the outcome. Outcomes are important. Of course, they are. However, if you become fixated on the outcome, it will work against you. That's because without focusing on the process, you will drift and get off track, making it harder to reach your weight-loss goal.

Make a lifestyle change instead of a life-changing transformation. What does this mean? People tend to get obsessed with making life changing transformations. Life-changing transformations usually fade away. Rather, get obsessed with the small daily lifestyle improvements that are needed to make the grand change possible.

Let me explain. Losing 50 pounds would be life-changing, right? However, drinking 10 glasses of pure water every day is a new lifestyle. You want to concentrate on the lifestyle you need to have and maintain so you can attain the healthy weight you seek.

21

WEIGHT LOSS IS A JIGSAW PUZZLE

"To solve your life's puzzle,
start with a clear purpose of the finished product."

– Darren Hardy

This chapter was inspired and based upon an episode of *Darren Daily* by Darren Hardy, *New York Times* best-selling author of *The Compound Effect* and world-renowned success mentor.

Healthy and sustainable weight loss is like putting together a jigsaw puzzle. When it comes to losing weight in a healthy and sustainable manner, not one size fits all. Each person is different. However, the guiding principles of putting a jigsaw puzzle together is very similar to achieving a healthy weight.

When they open a new 1,000-piece puzzle, most people dump the pieces onto the table. The whole task looks daunting and overwhelming. Looking at all the chaos, you might even question starting the project. That's the same feeling you might get when you start your weight-loss journey. The enormity of losing 10, 20, 30, 40, 50, or more pounds might confront you. This is why many people delay, procrastinate, and put off the idea of losing weight altogether.

However, you really want to do this jigsaw puzzle, so you dive-in and start flipping over all the pieces. Then you begin sorting them out by color into more manageable piles. This is how you should start your weight-loss journey – breaking your total weight-loss goal into smaller, more manageable increments. Instead of looking at shedding all 20, 30, 40, or more pounds, break it down into losing one to two pounds per week. This way it will not be too overwhelming.

The next step in putting together a jigsaw puzzle is to figure out what image you are creating. If you do not know how the final image is going to look, it will be nearly impossible to put it together. Yet, most people start their weight-loss journey without having a clear picture of what healthy eating and an improved lifestyle is supposed to look like. That's because they have never done it before. Just like starting a new jigsaw puzzle.

Another factor in putting together a jigsaw puzzle is that the end picture must be interesting. Let's face it; if you are going to put forth the time and effort to figure out the intricacies of the puzzle, you want to make certain you will enjoy the end result, which is the picture. Otherwise, you will lose interest and probably not finish it. This is the same for losing weight in a healthy and sustainable manner. You must believe the time and effort you are putting forth into improving your eating habits will give you more vitality, more energy, make you feel better, look better, and improve your overall health. Otherwise, why bother?

Here are some tips on how to put together a jigsaw puzzle and how to lose weight in a healthy and sustainable manner:

1. Build the border first.

The border creates the boundaries or framework to create order. In weight loss your border is your achievement system or process. This means you need to establish the framework you will operate within and the metrics to track your results. It's your Code of Honor, your Food Journal, your Accountability Partner, and the other tools we've examined in this book.

2. You can only work on one piece at a time.

You can do anything, just not everything. If you are attempting to get everything done, you most likely will be stressed along the way. With weight loss, you need to focus on improving one habit at a time. If you attempt to change everything at once, you will probably be overwhelmed and unable to improve or modify any of your eating habits. The next chapter has a great tool to help you do this.

3. Don't force a fit.

You might think certain pieces might go together. In fact, you want them to go together. However, they just don't fit quite right. If you force them together, it will ruin your entire puzzle. On the other hand, some pieces that don't seem to go together are a perfect fit. This applies to weight loss.

4. Don't force the issue.

If you are unable to do an intermittent fast for longer than 12 hours, don't force it. If you are initially unable to drink more than 64 ounces of pure water, don't force it. You want the process to fit you so that you will want to maintain it for your lifetime.

5. Sometimes you have to take a different perspective.

Every once in a while, you might want to get up and look at the puzzle from a different vantage point. This provides a different perspective of the big picture, which could help you see where another piece might fit. This applies to weight loss. You might need to track your eating habits to see if there is a piece missing in your process. It could be something as simple as reducing your portion sizes or eating a pear instead of an apple.

6. You are going to want to quit.

You will be tempted at some point in putting together the jigsaw puzzle to quit. Don't! As with weight loss, sometimes you get into a groove and you shed pounds quickly. It is exhilarating to have one success after another. However, when you hit a weight plateau, and you will, it is not as easy to continue. Frustration sets in. This is when you need to push through and realize that your body needs time to adjust to your new weight set point. This is when most people give up. They focused on the goals and not the process. Just keep moving forward one pound at a time.

7. The joy is in the journey, not the finish line.

Jigsaw puzzles are like goals because once you complete them, you need to start over again. To have fun putting another jigsaw puzzle together, you need to clear the old one and put it back in the box. The fun is in putting the puzzle together to see how the individual pieces fit together to form a picture. Similarly, healthy weight loss is a journey – it is a lifestyle. On your journey, though, there is no finish line. A diet has a finish line. It is like a sprint.

What then? Creating and maintaining a healthy lifestyle is like running a marathon without a finish line. You just keep going.

Life is like one big jigsaw puzzle because as soon as you die, your puzzle is completed, and your journey is over. Therefore, it is important to find joy in your journey and to have a life full of good health so you can enjoy it. Otherwise, a life full of illnesses, disease, and afflictions is not fun. There is no joy. Plus, you might become a burden to your family.

22

POSITION OF CONTROL – MASTERING THE ZORRO CIRCLE

"If you can't explain it simply, do it simply, design it simply, it is because you don't understand it well enough."

– Albert Einstein

What is the Zorro Circle, you might be wondering?
The Zorro Circle is a metaphor to limit your focus to master small, manageable goals, so later you can expand the scope of your ability and capability. In the movie *The Mask of Zorro,* Alejandro/Zorro (played by Antonio Banderas) is a broken man. That is because as a young man, his ambition to fight villains and right the injustices in the world far exceeded his knowledge and skill set. After many attempts and many failures, Alejandro, frustrated, feels disillusioned and powerless. He surrenders to alcohol, falls into a deep despair, and loses his confidence.

Fortunately for Alejandro, he meets a mentor, Don Diego (played by Anthony Hopkins), an aging sword master. It is Don Diego who helps Alejandro regain his confidence by helping him gain a sense of control, giving him back his focus, conviction, and perseverance.

When Alejandro first started, he had no focus and no sense of control. He wants to do too much too quickly. However, he does not know where to start. This is how many people who want to lose weight feel. They want to do too much too quickly. They are unaware of how to start to improve their eating habits. It can be daunting and overwhelming. Does this sound familiar?

There is a scene in the movie when Zorro's training commences. Don Diego places Alejandro in a small training circle. Don Diego tells him, *"This is called a training circle, a master's wheel. This circle will be your world, your whole life, until I tell you otherwise. There is nothing outside of it… As your skill with the sword improves, you will progress to a larger circle…"*

The small circle is for Alejandro to control. A simple path to follow, he must master what is inside the circle before he can expand it or move on to the next circle. This is what you must do to improve and master your daily eating habits. You must master one circle at a time. For instance, the first and most important daily eating habit you must master is to drink an adequate amount of pure water. This is the foundation of all healthy weight loss and healthy lifestyle.

Once Alejandro mastered control of that small circle, Don Diego slowly starts to expand his circle allowing him to attempt bigger and bigger feats, which one by one, Alenjadro achieves. Likewise, as you master drinking an adequate amount of pure water each day, then you can move on to the next circle, which is avoiding all processed and manufactured food products. And, once you mastered avoiding all processed and manufactured food products, then you move on to eating organic, whole, or holistic foods.

As Alejandro gained more confidence, he learned how to command his emotions and utilize his skills. None of Alejandro's achievements would have been possible had he not first been able to master that small circle. Similarly, what this means for you is it will be difficult, if not impossible, for you to achieve and maintain healthy weight loss if you do not first master being able to drink an adequate amount of pure water and control your emotions.

Before Alejandro mastered the small circle, he had no command over his emotions, no sense of his own skill, no real faith in his ability to accomplish a goal. And, worst of all, no feeling of control over his fate.

Do you feel this way too? That you have no control over your emotions, no sense of skill of how to eat healthy, or what it means to eat healthy, no real faith in your ability to accomplish your weight-loss goal? And no feeling of being able to control your daily eating habits to lose weight? Do you fail to make it to even the second Zorro circle (avoid processed and manufactured foods) because your cravings sabotage you? Let's talk about that.

CRAVINGS – Nothing more than cravings

Food cravings are your worst enemy for improving your eating behaviors. A food craving is an intense or uncontrollable urge for specific foods, stronger than normal hunger. Sugar cravings are a primary reason people have a hard time losing weight and eating healthy. Food cravings can be caused by many factors. Below are several things which might produce a craving.

Manufactured (not created by nature) and highly processed foods are a primary cause for cravings. Keep in mind that these edible products are scientifically engineered to optimize ***your*** cravings for them.

In other words, they are purposely designed to be addicting. When Lays says, "Betcha can't eat just one," it's not a dare. It is a fact. Eating a craved food less often, or not at all, may be more effective than eating a small portion of that food whenever you crave it. What's important to remember is that you might not be able to ever eat certain foods. As an example, in my situation I have not had a Pringle's potato chip, M&M, Snicker's, Hershey bar, Thin Mint Girl's Scouts cookie, and several other snack foods because I know if I have just one, I will not stop. I will keep wanting more and more of it. It is similar to an alcoholic having one drink. If they do, they will continue to have more.

An imbalance in the hunger hormones leptin and ghrelin might cause some people to experience more food cravings than others.

Lack of adequate quality sleep might disrupt your hormone levels in charge of regulating hunger, fullness, and sleep cycles which can intensify your cravings for food. This might explain why a lack of sufficient quality sleep causes many people, on average, to consume an extra 500 calories the next day.

Not drinking enough water to stay properly hydrated. Often a person who is thirsty thinks they are hungry when they actually need to drink more water.

A nutrient-deficient diet might be causing your cravings. If your diet is low in vegetables, fruits, nuts, berries, fiber, protein, healthy fats, and complex carbohydrates, it might be causing you to feel hungry or increase your cravings. Although you might be providing your body with a sufficient amount of calories, you might be depriving it of the right fuel, i.e., enough nutrients such as vitamins and minerals. What is important to remember is that all calories are not equal in nutritional value. A Hershey bar has no nutritional value compared to an apple. Yet, they have a similar number of calories. A lack of physical activity might cause you to have more food cravings, whereas doing something as simple as walking could reduce your cravings.

People who live in Blue Zones (areas of healthy longevity) do physical activity about every twenty minutes. You could get up from your chair and do some stretches or squats.

Stress can increase your cortisol levels. Cortisol is a hormone. High levels of this hormone have been linked to increased hunger, cravings for highly processed foods, and binge-eating behaviors. Look for other ways to decrease your stress levels such as deep breathing, meditation, or yoga.

Your eating environment can cause cravings for specific foods. As an example, popcorn and a movie or watching television. Or having a hot dog and either a soda or beer at a ballgame. Certain elements can trigger cravings for specific foods.

Your mood may play a role for cravings. How often do you or someone you know reach for the pint of ice cream if you or they are feeling sad or upset? Negative moods have been shown to increase a person's cravings for comfort foods.

Banish those cravings

Now that you are aware of some factors that might increase your cravings for certain foods, here are seven ways to stop cravings for sugar and unhealthy foods.

1. **Drink water**. As mentioned earlier, dehydration is mistaken for hunger or food cravings. What's important to remember is that 75 percent of the U.S. population is chronically dehydrated. If you have a sudden urge for a specific food, drink a large glass of water and wait a few minutes. Your craving might fade away because your body was thirsty.
2. **Eat more protein** because protein reduces cravings, helps you feel fuller and satisfied longer. Several studies of overweight people showed that increasing protein intake significantly reduced cravings and the desire to snack.
3. **Brush your teeth.** Research shows that a clean mouth tends to reduce cravings.
4. If you are having a craving for sugar, **eat a piece of fruit**. Having a piece of fruit such as an apple, pear, orange, or banana, might help you satisfy that sugar craving.
5. **Avoid *all* artificial sweeteners**. Studies have shown that artificial sweeteners may increase your craving for sweetness. This is one reason that a diet soda with artificial sweeteners causes weight gain.
6. **Talk with your accountability partner or success buddy.** Explain what you are going through and ask them for support.
7. **Read your affirmations/declarations**. It can be beneficial to carry your list of affirmations/declarations with you so that if you have a craving, you can use it for support.

8. **Physical activity**. Get up from your seat every 20 to 30 minutes and move. It could be a few stretches, a short walk, or some other physical activity.
9. **Take nutritional supplements.** Be consistent taking your supplements. If you do not take your supplements on a regular basis, it is almost the same as not taking them at all.

With your cravings defused, get back into the Zorro Circle

The lesson of the story of the Zorro circle is this: to achieve anything in life, you need to focus your efforts on small, manageable tasks, which once accomplished, gives a sense of control. This builds confidence. As your confidence grows, so will your desire to continue. By first limiting the extent of your weight-loss efforts, then watching those efforts have an intended effect, you gain knowledge and confidence to expand the circle, mastering larger and larger areas. Before long, you will change your daily eating habits, lose weight, feel better, improve your overall health, and want to do more.

I encounter clients who struggle to take charge of their own eating behaviors and lifestyles. The Zorro circle helps them take a simple path to accomplish their weight-loss success.

Your Zorro Circle:
The 9 Fundamental Principles for Healthy Weight Loss

1. Drink an adequate amount (64 ounces or more) of pure water each day
2. Avoid processed and manufactured foods, also known as edible products
3. Eat organic, holistic/whole foods, mostly plants
4. Eat slowly
5. Eat small portions.
6. Get adequate sleep.

7. Focus on the food you eat by eliminating distractions that can cause "mindless" eating.
8. Give your body 12 to 14 hours each day to digest and process the food you consume.

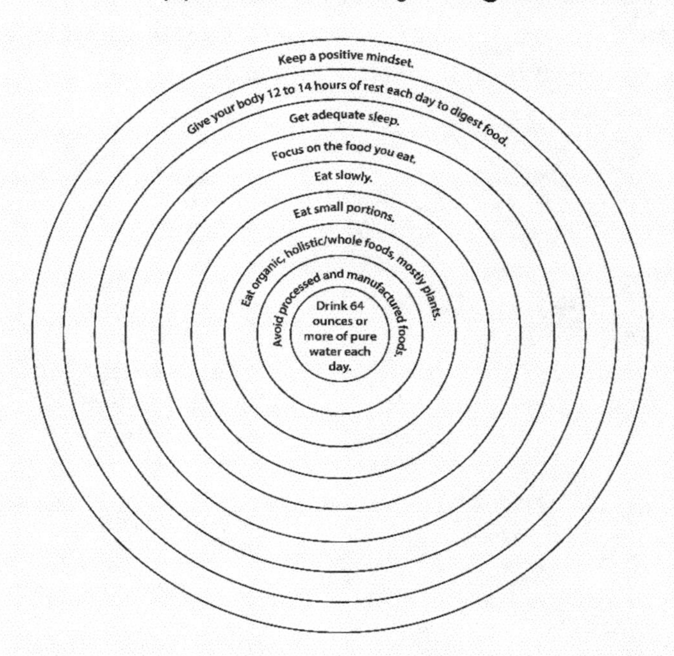

9. Keep a positive mindset by focusing on the foods you should eat that are healthy rather than the edible products you crave that are known to be unhealthy. What you focus on expands.

Knowing what to do to lose weight is a good start. Changing and improving daily habits is a key component of your weight-loss success and healthy weight management.

You don't need to modify all your bad habits at one time to significantly improve your life. Just as Alejandro had grand intentions, we all start with grand intentions to lose weight. However, we are overcome by the irresistible call of unhealthy foods and beverages. The instant gratification and comfort, not to mention the convenience, of these highly processed foods and artificially sweetened beverages overwhelms our sense and are hard to resist. This is why it is important to master a small circle, so we learn to control our emotions regarding food. Achieving your healthy and sustainable weight is possible, and you too can do it.

23

IF YOU WANT TO LIVE WELL, LIVE LIKE PEOPLE WHO LIVE LONG

"We do not need magic to change the world, we carry all the power we need ourselves already: we have the power to imagine better."

– J.K. Rowling
(Harry Potter creator)

People who live to a healthy age of 100 or older around the world are located in places known as Blue Zones. Dan Buettner, best-selling author of *The Blue Zones* and *The Blue Zones Kitchen* identified five areas around the world where people consistently live to a healthy age of 100 or more without taking supplements, pills, or anti-aging serums. What this means for you is if you want to live to a healthy age of 100 or older, live like those who've lived to be 100-plus years. Being healthy is more than just what we put into our mouths. It's a lifestyle, and eating is a part of that lifestyle.

The essence of having and keeping a healthy weight is to control or eliminate cravings, and reduce hunger, while adjusting your fullness level downward. What this means for you is you too can be on the better side of health through old values rather than the new creations of edible products.

I believe in improving the health of others. One common denominator of my clients - they want to have excellent health. My goal is to provide breakthrough health ideas to people who want to have and keep good health. A breakthrough idea does not necessarily mean a new idea. It can be an idea that is new to you.

Throughout this book I've done my best to provide you with principles and a process to implement them.

A principle is a proposition or value that is a guide for behavior or evaluation. In nature, it is a rule that has to be or usually is to be followed.

A process is a series of steps and decisions involved in the way something is completed. You may not realize it, but processes are everywhere and in every aspect of our leisure and work. A few examples of processes might include, however, not limited to how you prepare a meal, how you eat your meal, or even how you purchase the ingredients to prepare meals.

In my opinion, there are nine fundamental principles you need to have and keep a healthy weight. They have been identified and discussed all through this book. Doing them is the process. These are the steps to put the nine principles into action:

- Go Slow
- Take Small Steps
- Keep Moving Forward
- Focus on What to Eat Instead of What Not to Eat
- Celebrate Small Wins
- Trust the Process
- Get Results

Now you have the ingredients and direction to get a healthy weight and keep it. I wish you much success on your journey to have and maintain good health and to enjoy a higher quality of life than the average person. Be the health exception.

APPENDIX A

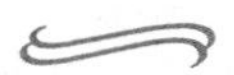

QUESTIONS TO PONDER

If you find yourself struggling with your weight-loss journey, take some time to reflect and answer the questions below. Write out your answers either in your food journal or on a piece of paper. You might find your solution in doing self-reflection.

What existing eating habits or behaviors do you need to expand?
For example,

- Could you drink more pure water?
- Could you eat more dietary fiber?
- Could you eat more vegetables?
- Can you eliminate processed and manufactured foods?

What poor eating habits or behaviors do you need to improve or stop?
For example,

- Could you stop drinking soda or diet soda?
- Could you stop going to the drive-thru, ordering pizza, picking up a bucket of fried chicken, or eating frozen microwaveable foods?
- Could you stop using ketchup as a condiment?
- Could you take more time to eat your meals instead of eating them while working or watching TV?

- Could you stop eating at least three hours before you go to sleep?

What new eating habits or behaviors do you need to start?

For example,

- Could you start using a salad plate instead of a dinner plate?
- Could you eat slower?
- Could you start drinking pure water?
- Could you start using a salad plate instead of a dinner plate to control your portions?

What are your top three modifications or improvements to your daily eating routine and how will you implement them?

1.
2.
3.

Tough Love Questions to ask yourself

STEP 1: Affirm your weight-loss goal.

- *Your goal is still to lose _____ pounds, right?*

STEP 2: Ask yourself if you think you are on or off track.

- *Are you on or off track to hitting your goal?*

Follow-up question:

- *If you are on track, how sure are you?* Or…
- *If you are on track, how do you know that for sure?*
- *If you are off track, what do you need to do to get back on track?*

STEP 3: When you self-confess, ask yourself,

- *"Why do you think that is?"*
- *Why do you think you are off track with your weight-loss plan?*

APPENDIX B

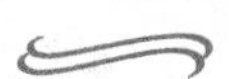

QUICK REFERENCE GUIDE

Throughout this book, you have been taught to be consistent with your improved eating behaviors as it relates to the food quality (the food choices) you consume, the portion sizes (how much you eat), how fast you eat, where you eat, and other issues.

This is a quick reference guide to remind you how to improve your eating habits.

Portions (How much should I eat?)

To help you determine the appropriate portion size for you and your body as it relates to protein, complex carbohydrates, and healthy fats, without using measuring cups, food scales, or other calorie-counting devices, use this quick reference guide:

- The palm of your hand determines the size of how much protein you should eat,
- Your fist determines the portion size of how much vegetables you should eat (although you can eat as many raw or steamed vegetables as you desire),
- Your cupped hand defines the portion size of complex carbohydrate you should consume, and

- Your thumb defines how much healthy fats you can consume

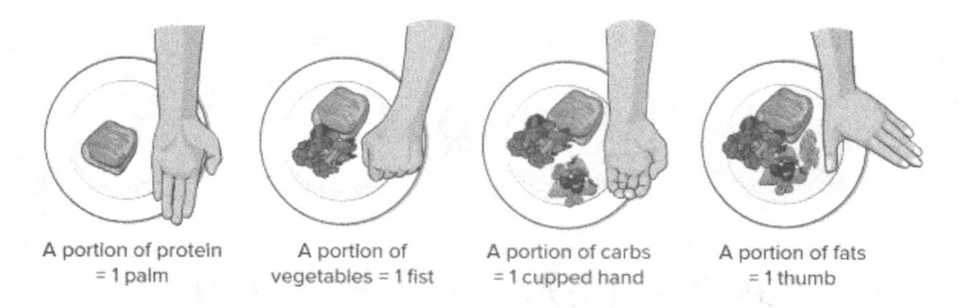

Counting Calories – No need to do it

For most people, counting calories does not work for delivering sustainable, healthy weight loss. Based on the experience of thousands of folks, there are several problems with counting calories. These include but are not limited to:

- The number of calories is meaningless to most people. If calories meant anything, people would avoid eating many of the meals listed on the menu at restaurants. When was the last time you paid attention to the calories shown on a menu?
- The calories do not distinguish between healthy foods and unhealthy foods. As an example, a regular size Hershey's chocolate bar has about 125 calories. An apple has about 100 calories. The apple provides more fiber and nutritional value than the Hershey's bar.
- The number of calories is often wrong. The number of calories in a food item is an estimate. That estimate can be off by as much as 20 percent.
- The number of calories does not factor in the impact of other eating behaviors such as where a person is eating, when a person is eating, or how fast a person is eating.
- Counting calories can create additional emotional, psychological, and mental issues for people.

- The point about counting calories is that it will not help you improve your eating behaviors and develop a healthier lifestyle. It might even thwart your relationship with food.

How often should I eat?

Contrary to popular belief, how often you eat does not matter very much depending on each person's situation. If you eat the right types of foods, in the right portions, in the right environment without distractions, then how often you eat becomes a matter of personal preference.

According to the Society of Sports Nutrition (ISSN), "The preponderance of the research suggests that increased meal frequency does not play a significant role decreasing body weight/weight composition." What this means for you is that how often or frequently you eat does not appear to matter when calories and macronutrients are the same.

Another common misconception is that smaller, more frequent meals will boost your metabolism. Several research studies have examined the impact of how often a person eats – from 1 to 17 meals – on a metabolic rate. What they found was it does not matter if you are a nibbler or a person who gorges. Of course, this assumes the food choices and amounts are the same. What this means for you is it doesn't matter if you want to have smaller more frequent meals throughout the day or eat one or two larger meals, so long as the food quality and amount are the same. Therefore, some people prefer to do an intermittent fast, while others prefer to do time restricted eating, and others prefer to limit their food intake to one meal per day. In other words, it is what works for you that is important.

Water Intake

Water is the ***most*** important aspect for excellent health. What is important to remember is that your body is composed of between 60 and 70 percent water. Thirst isn't usually realized until 2 to 3 percent of body water is lost. And, unfortunately, many people think they are hungry when they are, in fact, thirsty.

Researchers at the University of Utah found that dehydration of 2 to 3 percent can lower your metabolic rate. Participants in the study who drank eight to twelve 8-ounce glasses of water were adequately hydrated, had more energy, were able to concentrate better, and burned more calories than the participants who drank less than 64-ounces of water each day.

In addition, the researchers learned that "preloading" water had a direct positive impact on fat loss. Preloading refers to drinking 16-ounces of water 30-minutes before each meal. Those participants who preloaded water before each meal lost five times more weight than those who pre-loaded only once per day or not at all over the course of 12 weeks.

In a separate study done by Virginia Tech and published in the journal of *Obesity,* participants who combined water preloading with a reduced caloric intake lost 64 percent more fat than those who followed the same reduced caloric intake without the water preload.

What this means for you is that drinking an adequate amount of water is extremely important to your overall health, metabolism, performance, and has direct beneficial correlation to fat loss.

- Drinking 16 ounces of water before each meal and between 96 and 128 ounces each day is critical to effective and sustainable weight loss.

Sleep – it has a tremendous impact on your weight loss efforts.

Lack of sleep will affect your weight loss efforts. Researchers from the University of Chicago and the University of Wisconsin conducted a study to determine if sleep deprivation had an impact on a reduced-calorie diet. What they found was startling. Participants who slept 5.5 hours per night lost 55 percent less fat and burned 60 percent more muscle mass than those who slept 8.5 hours. This demonstrates that lack of sleep can make a significant impact on your weight loss efforts.

Losing muscle mass is not healthy. Further, lack of adequate sleep, that is 8 hours or more, in addition to hampering your weight loss journey can have negative health side effects such as:

- Decreased carbohydrate tolerance
- Decreased insulin sensitivity
- Elevated levels of cortisol (a stress hormone)
- Lower levels of leptin (a fat-burning hormone)
- Higher levels of ghrelin (a hunger hormone)
- Increased hunger and appetite
- Reduced muscle recovery

Perhaps making a few small adjustments to the behaviors mentioned above can help you improve your daily eating habits and help you along your weight-loss journey while improving your overall health.

APPENDIX C

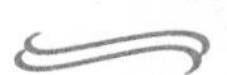

THE OVERWEIGHT PERSON'S BEST FRIEND QUOTES

The Best of David Medansky

When you eat for health, your weight-loss journey will take care of itself. Never go on a diet. Instead, change your diet. What this means for you is simply eat more foods that promote health and fewer manufactured and processed foods aka "Edible Products" that promote disease.

Your Fat is the Real "F" Bomb.

If we put off until tomorrow what we can do today, and tomorrow never comes, that means we will never do what needs to be done.

You will be more disappointed that you didn't eat healthier and put the proper fuel in your body 20 years from now than if you start today.

If you want to be thinner, don't listen to overweight people.

Intention is the first step to reducing weight. Commitment is the second step. The third step is action. Celebrate achieving small weight reduction goals is the fourth step. Follow through is the fifth step.

What shapes our weight reduction success are the questions we ask, the questions we refuse to ask, and the questions we never think to ask. Often, we don't know what we don't know.

Stay committed to reducing weight and you will succeed achieving a healthy weight and maintaining it.

If you keep on doing what you've been doing to lose weight and it's not working, you'll keep on failing, so don't be surprised!

We can't always be perfect. However, we can strive to improve each day. I no longer listen to what people tell me about their diet; I just watch what they eat.

It's not what you say you're going to do that defines you, it's what you do that defines who you are.

I could never find the right weight-loss program that would provide healthy and sustainable results, so I created it myself.

The battle with maintaining a healthy weight dictates that it must be fought every day.

Be prepared each day to confront your self-sabotage along your weight-loss journey.

When it comes to losing weight, stick to the simple and execute.

Simply eat more foods that promote health and fewer foods – aka 'Edible Products' – that promote disease.

Always ask yourself if what you are eating is getting you closer to your healthy weight-loss goals.

Shatter the beliefs you've been told about weight loss because diets are designed to fail.

Being healthy is not eating what most people are consuming as food.

The fundamentals of excellent health are simple. Getting yourself to do them is the difficult part.

Committing yourself to permanent improvements to your daily eating habits is the only way to lose weight in a healthy manner and keep it off.

There is more than one path to losing weight. Make sure you are on the right path for you.

In the absence of clear weight-loss guidelines, people drift. When you drift you follow your own beliefs, which may or may not be accurate.

You can never own your weight-loss success. You can only rent it. And the rent is due every day in the form of the food and beverage choices you choose to eat and drink.

Don't quit. Just because you don't see results immediately, don't give up. You may not see changes, however, every smart choice you make is affecting you in ways you'd never imagine. It is the smallest, seemingly inconsequential changes done consistently over time that can make the biggest difference to successfully reduce weight and keep it off.

All foods are an edible product. However, not all edible products are food. Food provides nutritious fuel for your body. An edible product merely fills your belly with toxic chemicals, so you are not hungry.

Conventional diets do not work. They make you miserable, and the word "Diet" has "Die" in it.

It is not your fault you did not lose weight on that diet. The diet is to blame. You did not fail the diet. The diet failed you.

For your weight-loss journey to succeed, you must find a way to remove all thinking, all discipline, and all willpower from the equation. If you need to rely on that, you're screwed.

There is no miraculous fruit, berry, nut, vegetable, or supplement to permanently lose weight. If there was, we'd all be thinner.

Hopefully, you understand that wanting, wishing, hoping, or praying to lose weight is not going to produce results.

On your weight-loss journey, you will be off track some of the time. That is because old habits are hard to break, and new habits are difficult to create. What is important to remember is the key to weight-loss success is to keep correcting your eating behaviors to put you back on track.

You will never change your weight and improve your health until you change your daily eating habits. The secret of your weight-loss success is found in your daily eating routines.

Keep this in mind; your weight is based 100 percent on what you eat and drink. Exercise is for fitness and overall health and wellness.

People always confuse weight loss with exercising. You can shed weight without exercising. However, you can never exercise enough to overcome poor eating habits.

Let's face it; it is easier to keep eating the same unhealthy fast foods and snacking on junk food than it is to prepare healthy, nutritious meals and snacks.

So many people are overweight that we lose perspective. You see so many other people heavier than you that you think you are fine because you are thinner. You're wrong. You're both overweight.

Your clothes will tell you everything about being thinner.

When you stop making excuses for why you are overweight, you will start to see results.

When it comes to eating healthy and making better food choices, understand that you can. The question is: will you?

A weight-loss goal without a proven process or system is just wishful thinking.

Stop pointing fingers saying you are not the weight you want to be because of him, her, or anybody. You choose what to put into your mouth. You decide what you are going to eat, where you are going to eat, when you are going to eat, and how fast you will eat. Until you make a commitment to improve your eating habits, you are never going to shed those excess pounds. You are better than that!

To achieve healthy sustainable weight loss, you will have to do something you don't want to do, something that will take effort and time. And you will constantly be pushed against the walls of your comfort zone.

The analogy of losing weight is similar to running a sprint versus running a marathon. A diet is a sprint. It has a finish line. Ninety percent of those who lose weight by dieting regain it. That's because they revert back to their old habits. However, those who shed weight by improving their lifestyle and eating habits keep the weight off because it is like running a marathon, except there is no finish line. You just keep going and going.

The biggest regret people have about losing weight is not starting a year earlier. The second biggest regret about attaining a healthy weight is not starting now.

With respect to weight reduction, there are three types of people: 1) those who think about losing weight, 2) those who talk endlessly about losing weight and do nothing, and 3) those who act to reduce weight. Which one are you?

If you make a conscious decision, you can eat slower. Yes, you can adapt and modify your eating behaviors.

A small taste of victory will build your confidence and increase your desire to do more to improve your eating habits and reduce weight. Even shedding two or three pounds the first few weeks is a victory.

It has been scientifically proven that the size of your dinnerware affects your behavior for how much food you consume. Consider this: If you increase your caloric intake by just 50 calories per day because you're eating more than you should, you will gain an additional five pounds within one year. This is how weight creeps up on us. It's gradual over a long period of time. Imagine reversing that trend and eating less simply by using a smaller plate, such as a salad plate instead of a dinner plate. You'd most likely reduce your caloric intake by 50 calories per day. Which means that over time, you'd get rid of extra weight.

You want to lose weight, right? I don't believe anyone wakes up in the morning wanting to be overweight, unhealthy, have low energy, and have low self-confidence. We all want to have more vitality and good health.

So, what keeps you from improving your eating habits and losing weight? Think positively. Watch your thoughts. Watch your words. They have impact. You are not making a sacrifice by avoiding certain foods. You are making a choice. You are not depriving yourself of anything, i.e., sweets, ice cream, cookies, cake, pie, etc. You are making a choice.

Do you want to reduce weight and improve your eating habits or not? If so, what are you willing to improve and change to make it happen? We can all agree nothing about your weight will change if you are not willing to do something different.

Have you attempted to lose weight before only to have someone tell you, *"Have just one. It won't kill you."* Or *"one cookie won't hurt you."* No, it won't hurt you. No, it won't kill you. However, it will prevent you from accomplishing your goal of getting rid of your extra weight.

We are all mentally weak when it comes to shedding weight.

Our mind is what sabotages us the most when it comes to weight loss.

The epic battle of getting rid of your unwanted weight will be won defeating your own mind.

When it comes to losing weight, the toughest person to negotiate with is yourself.

If you find yourself thinking or engaging in any negative self-talk – stop it.

To successfully lose weight and maintain a healthy body weight for life, you will need to fix the negative self-talk you have been engaging in.

Every person who has attempted to lose weight knows that battle. It is the self-talk, or management of it, that will get you through difficult times, or cause you to succumb.

No one is perfect. If you do overindulge, don't beat yourself up over it. Just keep moving forward.

You're better than that! So, keep moving forward.

People without a support team or someone to hold them accountable tend to give up on weight-reduction programs. It is difficult to have a spouse or significant other eating pizza, pasta, or desserts while you're attempting to improve your eating habits. Most people, with few exceptions, need to have someone to check in with to keep them accountable and stay on track.

Weight loss happens when you make small, seemingly inconsequential decisions to the foods you consume. If you are making bad decisions, take away your choices. Decide at the beginning of the day those foods you will eat. Focus on the positive. Avoid focusing on those foods that you should not eat.

In the absence of clear weight-loss guidelines, people drift. When you drift, you follow your own beliefs, which may or may not be accurate.

Commitment, a burning desire, focus, and consistent action are the magical ingredients necessary for your successful weight-loss journey to be realized.

What we don't realize is some people, like me, had to go through the experience of gaining and losing weight to get to where they are in life as it relates to weight. Let me explain. Like many of you, I wasn't always overweight. I was fit and trim. However, as with many of you, life happened. Before I realized it, I had gained a lot of weight. I had to experience the failure of gaining weight to experience the success of reducing weight.

There are many ways to lose weight and keep it off. You only need to figure out the one way for you to reduce weight in a healthy manner that you can sustain.

Big mistakes generally start as small errors. Gaining weight starts by making choices to eat differently. It's more convenient to pick up food at a drive-thru than prepare a meal at home. We're tired, hungry, and we become complacent. Over time, these tiny choices accumulate and show on our waistline or with us ending up with a medical ailment.

When we maintain our integrity to improve our eating habits, we pay attention to the choices we make each day. The nearer we live to the source of health the more health we shall receive.

When confronted with making a mistake while attempting to reduce weight, do you pull back, retreat? Or do you rise to the challenge, figure out a way to overcome the obstacle preventing your weight loss, and move forward?

People would rather eat that pizza every Saturday night than think about how much weight they will gain in a year by doing so.

Lack of consistency will derail your weight-loss success. The start and stop process of diets kills the progress of your own weight-loss pursuit and permanent results.

Consistency is the single most important predictor of weight-loss success. You can accomplish what seems incredible, extraordinary results in short spurts. However, if it is not continued, it eventually is all for nothing. Why do you think more than 90 percent of those who go on a diet to lose weight fail?

With respect to weight loss, you want a system instead of a goal. Losing 10, 15, 20, 30 or more pounds is a goal. Learning to eat right is a system. Having a goal is not going to help you lose weight. The system to achieve the goal is what you want to focus your energy on. The goal is the destination. The system is the map to guide you on your journey.

When it comes to weight loss, systems will always trump goals. Whatever your weight-loss or fitness goals might be, make sure you have a system to achieve your goal.

Healthy and sustainable weight loss is about getting you to do what you know needs to be done consistently and permanently. After all, most of us know what to do when it comes to eating healthy. We just don't do it. The greatest threat to achieving and maintaining weight-loss success is not failure, it is boredom.

The journey to achieving and maintaining weight-loss success is very mundane and unexciting because you are eating mostly the same foods over and over. However, it is punctuated by flash moments of extreme excitement when the scale reads a certain number, or you have a smaller clothes size.

Let's face it, diets tend to be extreme, temporary, hard to stick with, and potentially dangerous to your health.

Saying "I'm on a diet" carries an assumed message that it is something you will eventually stop doing and go off of.

We all have good intentions to lose weight. You might have tried a diet and failed and tried another and failed again. When this happens, admit you're stuck. Ask for support. Ask someone to keep you accountable.

If you are attempting to lose weight, it's not what you do when people are watching, it's what you do in private when no one is watching. Keep in mind what you do in private, you wear in public.

Our instinctive reaction when we "cheat" on our weight-loss journey is to shift blame rather than accept responsibility for our actions and learn from it. It is more empowering for you to accept your role in choosing to indulge, learn from your setback, and move on.

Gaining weight starts by making choices to eat differently. It is more convenient to pick up food at a drive-thru, order a pizza, get a bucket of fried chicken with sides than to prepare a meal at home. You are tired, hungry, and you become complacent. Over time, these small, seemingly inconsequential choices accumulate and show on our waistline or cause a medical ailment, debilitating illness, or disease.

Your weight-loss history does not predict your future. You have options. When confronted with making a mistake while attempting to reduce weight, do you pull back, retreat?

Being overweight is failure. It is a failure of not drinking enough pure water and eating healthier. It is failure by choosing to eat processed and manufactured groceries than to eat whole, holistic, and real foods. A mistake can teach you, through analysis and feedback, what's working and what's not working.

Are you inspired by others who are successfully dropping weight? Does that inspire you to do the same? If not, why not? What will inspire and motivate you to do something?

APPENDIX D

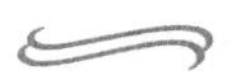

AFFIRMATIONS – DECLARATIONS

- I begin the day expecting amazing things.
- I begin the day being grateful for what I have and what I will receive.
- I begin the day open to receiving new ideas, new information, and new connections.
- I begin the day letting go of what's not serving me. Some refer to this as "bless and release."
- I begin the day being a positive influence on others.
- I am whole, perfect, strong, powerful, loving, harmonious, grateful, confident, healthy, and happy. I am love. I am compassionate. I am good fortune. I am positive energy flowing to the higher good.
- Napoleon Hill began his day reciting, "O Divine Providence, I ask not for more riches, [instead, I ask for] more wisdom with which to make wiser use of the riches you gave me at birth, consisting in the power to control and direct my own mind to whatever ends I desire."
- I am slim and fit.
- I am CONFIDENT!
- I am strong and beautiful at my healthy weight.

- I am retaining my ideal weight.
- I eat proper portions. I enjoy using a salad plate instead of a dinner plate.
- I am an inspiration to others to reduce weight. If I can do it, others can too!
- I am living a healthy lifestyle and improve each day.
- My body is a fat-burning machine.
- I am accountable for my choices.
- I use creative alternatives to keep focused and committed to keeping my weight-reduction goals.
- I am resolved to sustaining my reduced weight in a healthy manner.
- I use positive words with myself and others.
- My healthy eating habits make me smile with pride.
- I allow myself to make food choices and decisions for my higher good regardless of what others might say or think.
- I look and feel terrific. I love my body.
- I am grateful for being thin and fit.
- I am grateful for being able to make better food choices.
- I am worry free, stress free, and drama free.
- I am resolved to maintaining my reduced weight in a healthy manner.
- I encourage myself with positive self-talk.

RECOMMENDED READS:

Sugar Blues by William Dufty

Food Sanity by David Friedman, N.D., D.C.

If Not Now, When? By David Medansky

How to Fight FATflammation! By Lori Shemek, Ph.D., CNC

The Blue Zones by Dan Buettner

Feeding You Lies by Vani Hari

The Blues Zones Kitchen by Dan Buettner

The Compound Effect by Darren Hardy

The Traveler's Gift by Andy Andrews

Bright Line Eating by Susan Pierce Thompson

Live Young Forever by Jack LaLanne and all Jack LaLanne Books

Bragg Healthy Lifestyle by Paul Bragg and all of Paul and Patricia Bragg Books

ACKNOWLEDGEMENT

The Universe was smiling down upon me when Darren Hardy entered my life and inspired me to write this book.

If you've read *The Compound Effect*, *The Entrepreneur Roller Coaster*, or *Living Your Best Year Ever*, you know that this New York Times best-selling author has abundant wisdom and knowledge to share. I am grateful and blessed that he has shared some of that knowledge with me.

Darren is a world-renowned success mentor to leaders and high-performing achievers. He's a keynote speaker, advisor, a former publisher of *SUCCESS* magazine, and founder of *DarrenDaily*, an online daily video blog with one big idea delivered in under five minutes to give an advantage to having a successful day.

He's created courses including eFastPass, Insane Productivity, Jumpstart, and a Hero's Journey. I am so grateful for having had the opportunity to participate in these courses and programs. I made many references to Darren throughout this book because his mentoring and inspiration continued to bubble up into new ideas as I created *Break the Chains of Dieting*. I appreciate Darren Hardy and his A-Team for making a positive impact on my life and the lives of others.

ABOUT THE AUTHOR

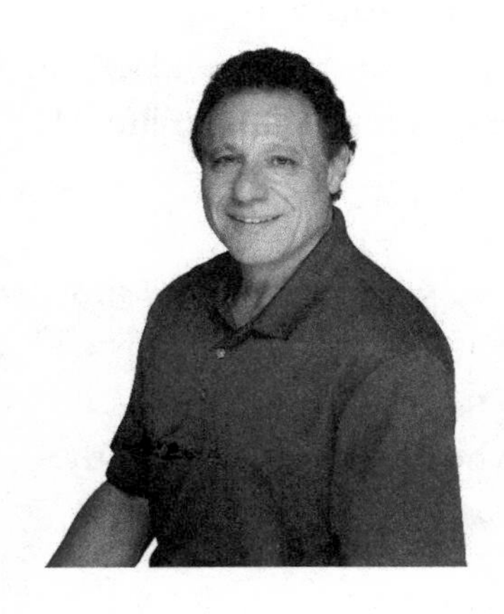

David Medansky, The Overweight Person's Best Friend, is a former divorce attorney, an international award-winning best-selling author, and Founder of 21-Day Jumpstart Weight Loss Program.

People hire David to teach them how to break through their resistance to improve their eating habits so they can lose weight, have more energy, feel better, look better, and enhance their overall health without going on a diet.

Diets tend to be extreme, temporary, hard to stick with, and potentially harmful. David teaches people how to stop wasting money on FAD (Fat and Desperate) diets because diets are designed to fail.

David struggled with his own weight issues until July of 2016 when his doctor told him to lose weight or find a new doctor. He understands your frustrations. David found a way to shed 50 pounds, almost 25 percent of his total body weight. Now he wants to teach you how to eat healthier so you can have more energy, feel better, and improve your overall health without having to order special meals or, purchase diet supplements or products, without having to count calories and without having to follow a specific exercise program.

If you're struggling to reduce weight or keep it off, David's *9 Fundamental Must Have Principles for Healthy Weight Loss* is a good place to start your weight loss journey.

You can learn more at www.breakthedietchains.com

Thank you for investing in yourself and in this book. If you have found value in this book, if it has helped you in any way, please leave an honest review. In addition, please consider giving a copy to five people whom you care about and for whom you want to have better health. The recipients could be relatives, friends, team members, vendors, or someone you would like to make a discernable difference in their life. My goal is to make a positive impact in the lives of millions of people. To do that, I need your help.

I promise you in the long run it will be you who benefits the most. Your helping someone else find ideas to improve their eating habits and improve their overall health could alter the course of their life…possibly save someone's life. Because without you who gives it to them, they might never have found *Break the Chains of Dieting.*

Write down five people you will give a copy of this book to:

____

____

____

____

____

Thank you for doing this for me.
I wish you good HEALTH above all else.

David Medansky
The Overweight Person's Best Friend

If what you have read, resonates with you –
I would love for you to leave an honest review on
Amazon or Goodreads

SPECIAL INVITATION

Would you like help to improve your eating habits, health, and other areas of your life? Do you need help being held accountable to reach your goals?

Then you have come to the right place.

I'd like to introduce you to Oola. Oola exists to make the world better by providing a structure that helps individuals create a life of balance, growth and purpose. It is the only lifestyle framework that combines an eLearning platform with a support system that encourages community and accountability.

Oola focuses on a life that is balanced in the 7 key areas: Fitness, Finance, Family, Field, Faith, Friends, and Fun.

Founded in 1997 by international best-selling authors, work-life balance experts, and holistic health care providers, Oola provides a simple, easy-to-follow lifestyle framework designed to lead you, step by step, to a life of less stress, more personal growth, and a clearer path toward living your unique purpose. Since the first copy of the blockbuster book, ***Oola: Find Balance in an Unbalanced World***, rolled off the presses, the Oola lifestyle has become a global phenomenon with over a million followers actively creating their best lives.

To learn more about Oola go to
https://myoola.oolalife.com/DavidMedansky
or https://bit.ly/2XALrud